LEGUMES

The Super Foods That Should Be Regulars on Your Plate

LEGUMES

The Super Foods That Should Be Regulars on Your Plate

Swarna Moldanado, Ph.D.

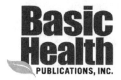

Basic
Health
PUBLICATIONS, INC.

The information contained in this book is based upon the research and personal and professional experiences of the author. It is not intended as a substitute for consulting with your physician or other healthcare provider. Any attempt to diagnose and treat an illness should be done under the direction of a healthcare professional.

The publisher does not advocate the use of any particular healthcare protocol but believes the information in this book should be available to the public. The publisher and author are not responsible for any adverse effects or consequences resulting from the use of the suggestions, preparations, or procedures discussed in this book. Should the reader have any questions concerning the appropriateness of any procedures or preparation mentioned, the author and the publisher strongly suggest consulting a professional healthcare advisor.

Basic Health Publications, Inc.
28812 Top of the World Drive
Laguna Beach, CA 92651
949-715-7327 • www.basichealthpub.com

Library of Congress Cataloging-in-Publication Data is available
through the Library of Congress.

Interior photos copyright Can Stock Photo.

Editor: Roberta W. Waddell
Typesetting/Book design: Gary A. Rosenberg
Cover design: Mike Stromberg

Printed in the United States of America

10   9   8   7   6   5   4   3   2   1

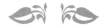

Contents

Acknowledgments, vii

Preface, ix

Introduction, 1

1. Legume Consumption—A Historical Perspective, 5

2. The Food Value of Legumes, 13

3. Straight Talk on Buzzwords, 19

4. Health Implications of Changes in the Traditional Diet of Selected Countries, 31

5. Most Commonly Eaten Legumes in the U.S. and Around the World, 61

6. Cooking, Sprouting, and Storing Legumes, 87

7. Recipes, 93

Summary, 147

References, 151

Recommended Reading, 153

Index, 157

About the Author, 165

To Alex,
for his abiding faith in me.

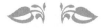

Acknowledgments

I want to express my heartfelt gratitude to my publisher Norman Goldfind for accepting my work. I also owe my thanks to him for assigning Bobby Waddell as my editor. Bobby is a master of her craft, and her attention to detail is awe-inspiring. I feel fortunate to have had her as my editor. My thanks to Mike Stromberg for his ingenuity in designing the book cover, and to Gary Rosenberg for undertaking the tedious task of making the illustrations fit the text perfectly. Finally, my special thanks go to my new friend Mary McVey Gill for reading the introductory sections and offering me her suggestions from which I benefited.

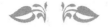

Preface

While I was growing up in India, legumes were a regular part of my diet. I don't remember when one kind of legume or another was not part of a meal, beginning with breakfast. Although we were not vegetarians as a family, and ate meat, poultry, and fish a few times a week, grains, legumes, and vegetables were the dominant part of our diet. But that changed when I emigrated to the U.S. Here my plate was filled more with meat or meat products, less with grains and vegetables, and rarely with legumes. This was not a conscious choice on my part, but came about because of what was served in the places I ate, such as campus cafeterias.

At first, I did not pay much attention to the missing familiar elements, like legumes, but once I started preparing my own meals, I realized what I had been missing in my American diet and started adding them back again. Chief among them were dry beans, peas, and lentils. Over the years, I noticed that, while the typical American diet often included fresh green beans and peas, it rarely contained dry beans, peas, and lentils.

As a nurse educator with a background in public health, I often talked about the importance of a healthful diet for preventing disease and promoting health. For decades, people have known that the large amounts of saturated fat contained mainly in meat, poultry, and other animal products is unhealthy, and that the unsaturated fat contained mainly in plant-based foods, is healthy. Yet, like much of the diet in

Western Europe, the standard American diet (SAD) consists of an abundance of calorie-dense, high-fat, animal-based foods, and an insufficient amount of low-fat, high-fiber, plant-based foods. This is despite the United States Department of Agriculture's recommendation to eat five to seven servings of fruits and vegetables daily, and at least three cups of legumes a week, or half a cup of cooked legumes each day.

My initial research into why there was a lack of enthusiasm for legumes in the American diet was quite revealing. The reasons included many prevailing misconceptions and inaccuracies about legumes as a food. Recognizing that a first step in facilitating any change in behavior, including eating behavior, is to make accurate, credible information available, I expanded my research to include learning about legume-based diets in selected countries around the world. My purpose was to learn how the traditional legume-based diets impacted health and disease in those countries. This book is the result of that quest, and fulfills my desire to share my findings with a broader audience.

Although this is not a book on weight loss, the steadily rising rates of overweight and obesity in the U.S., and the chronic diseases attributable to marked overweight were also factors prompting me to write this book.

The book is divided into seven main chapters and a summary, followed by the back matter. Chapter 1 deals with a global evolutionary account of dry beans, peas, and lentils in the human diet. Chapter 2 details the value and benefits of legumes as food. Because nutrition and health literature is fraught with buzzwords, Chapter 3 is devoted to providing factual descriptions of terms that are most frequently heard. Chapter 4 is a compilation of findings from several studies on diet and the implications for health and disease in selected countries over time. Chapter 5 discusses the most commonly consumed legumes around the world. Chapter 6 outlines methods of preparing, cooking, and sprouting legumes, and Chapter 7 provides sample recipes for cooking with legumes. The Summary, References, Recommended Reading, and an Index finish out the book.

—S.M

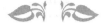

Introduction

It is no secret that two out of three Americans are overweight and two out of five are obese, the latter term generally defined as being 30 percent or more over the ideal body weight. This is in spite of the collective obsession about being thin. As a nation, Americans have not always been fat, so why are they now succumbing to this burgeoning health problem?

A partial answer may be found in the fact that the current environment is inundated with unhealthy foods that not only lead to weight gain, but also lay the foundation for chronic diseases, such as heart disease, certain cancers, and adult-onset diabetes. Conversely, some foods that provide good nutrients in abundance to help people stay lean and healthy for the long run remain below the radar and don't get the attention they deserve. Legumes undoubtedly belong to the latter category, and for a variety of reasons they have been undervalued, underconsumed, and even maligned as a food.

In this book, the word *legume* is used to refer to dry beans, peas, and lentils, although technically the term can refer to podded vegetables in general. Botanically, legumes are seeds of plants belonging to the family *Leguminosae*, which is one of the three largest families of flowering plants. Legumes have been cultivated and consumed for thousands of years in many parts of the world, and are considered super foods. What makes them super foods? Although, to date, there does not seem to be an agreed-upon or universally accepted definition of what super foods are, those foods generally referred to as super foods, such as almonds, avocados, bananas, blueberries, legumes, oats, pomegranates, pumpkins, walnuts, and wild-caught salmon, share some attributes. They are rich in vitamins and minerals, contain generous amounts of soluble and insoluble fiber (both associated with significant health benefits), have little or no saturated fat, and are generally low in calories. Naturally, any food that has these qualities belongs in a class above foods that lack one or more of these health-promoting and disease-preventing attributes.

Legumes as a group not only possess all the nutritional qualities mentioned above, but are also high in protein. They are deficient in a sufficient quantity of one essential amino acid to make them a *complete* protein, but the missing amino acid can be obtained from a complementary food, such as a grain, and the combination makes them a complete protein. Legumes as a source of protein are particularly important in plant-based diets. The 2010 *Dietary Guidelines for Americans*, developed by the U.S. Department of Health and Human Services (USDHHS) and the U.S. Department of Agriculture (USDA) recommend three cups of legumes per week, or half a cup of cooked legumes on a daily basis. This recommendation is based on empirical data drawn from studies that have shown that eating at least 100 grams of legumes per week is associated with many health benefits.

In a twenty-five-year study that examined food-intake patterns and risk of death from coronary heart disease, researchers followed more than 16,000 middle-aged men in the U.S., Finland, Greece, Italy, Japan, the Netherlands, and the former Yugoslavia.

The typical food patterns found were:

- Higher consumption of dairy products in Northern Europe;

- Higher consumption of meat in the U.S.;

- Higher consumption of vegetables, legumes, fish, and wine in Southern Europe; and

- Higher consumption of cereals, soy products, and fish in Japan.

When researchers examined the data in relation to the risk of death from heart disease, they found that legumes were associated with an 82-percent reduction in risk of death from coronary heart disease.

There is another beneficial attribute of legumes, although not derived from *eating* them, namely their ability to absorb nitrogen from the air and convert it into nitrates in the soil, a process referred to as *nitrogen-fixation,* which serves as a natural fertilizer. Legume plants accomplish this useful function with the aid of the *rhizobium* bacteria they harbor within their plant-root nodules. Legume crops build nitrogen levels in the soil as they grow, and benefits from the enhanced soil are achieved through crop rotations (inter-cropping) with non-nitrogen-fixing cereal grains. Since antiquity, the historical crop rotation of beans and maize (corn) in native cultures has capitalized on this characteristic property of legumes to produce higher yields of corn.

Why aren't legumes figuring as prominently in the American diet as they are in other regions of the world? The obvious explanation for the difference lies in the dietary patterns of the respective regions. Legumes like chickpeas appear in varied forms in the Mediterranean diet. A variety of dry beans constitute an important part of the South American diet. A wide variety of dry beans and lentils are a part of the daily diet across all regions of India. In other regions of Asia, people have found multiple creative ways to consume the much-touted soybean. The high content and quality of protein in soybean nearly matches animal protein. Although United States is one of the top producers of soybean, the legume is primarily consumed as an ingredient of many processed foods here.

A second reason for the scant consumption of legumes by Americans is the inconvenience associated with their preparation and cooking. Dry beans, except for lentils, need to be soaked in water for several hours before cooking and thus require advance planning prior to meal preparation. While many canned legumes come pre-cooked, they frequently contain significant amounts of salt and other additives. For convenience, raw legumes cannot compete with the timesaving processed and prepackaged foods that can go directly from the refrigerator or freezer to the oven or stovetop, a much-appreciated benefit in today's busy households.

A third reason for the lack of enthusiasm for legumes, especially among Americans, has to do with long-held stereotypes and attitudes toward legumes. They are often considered a poor man's food that does not lend itself to culinary creativity. Expressions that denigrate beans, such as *he doesn't know beans* about, used to indicate that someone is not well informed on a subject. And the expressions *don't amount to a hill of beans* when referring to worthless things, or nick-naming one of the oldest cities in the Northeastern United States *Beantown* don't help either.

Then, too, there's the fact that dry peas, beans, and lentils don't come in attractive packages with glossy, colorful pictures on the packages. In short, to many Americans, raw legumes don't appear to be foods that could be turned into interesting or tasty dishes.

Perhaps the most important overall reason for an inadequate consumption of legumes in the United States is the insufficient attention given them as nutritious, healthful, lean-protein, and high-fiber foods by American nutritional and dietary groups. Despite being recommended in the *Dietary Guidelines for Americans*, released annually by the U.S. Departments of Health and Human Services, and Agriculture, legumes have not caught on as a nutritious and healthful food with the general public. Given their good taste, health-promoting and disease-preventing attributes, ready availability, and low cost, legumes need to be embraced as the super foods they are, deserving of a more frequent presence on the American plate.

The following chapters delve into the many nutritional and health benefits of legumes to help readers think of them not just as occasional or exotic foods, but as nutritious, healthful, and tasty components of a well-balanced diet.

✦ 1 ✦

Legume Consumption— A Historical Perspective

Leguminous plants were among the first crops grown by human beings. The term legume is derived from the Latin word legumen, which means "to gather" in its verb form legere. Beans were among the first and most important foods to be gathered, and humans gathered wild legumes long before they domesticated them. Tens of thousands of years ago, for example, fava beans and chickpeas were food for hunter-gatherers in Central Asia and the Himalayan foothills. They were gradually cultivated in much of Asia, the Middle East, and Egypt, and became staples in many diets. The Phoenicians are believed to have carried the chickpea to the Western end of Europe, where it became entrenched in the diet of Iberians and continues to occupy an important place in their diet to this day. The lentil, the pea, and the broad bean can all be traced to present-day Afghanistan, Northwestern India, Tadzhikistan, Uzbekistan, and Western China. The American common bean and the lima bean are both said to have originated in the regions of Southern Mexico and Central America. The historical documents and reports kept by the Spanish explorers reveal that varieties of the common bean were grown by Native Americans as far South as Chile and Argentina, and as far North as the valleys of the St. Lawrence and upper Missouri rivers. The common bean further developed into other varieties, such as the black bean, great Northern bean, kidney bean, navy bean, pinto bean, and white bean.

The history of legumes goes back to the Neolithic era, when

humans transitioned from being hunter-gatherers to producing food through their own work. Early civilizations in Asia, the Americas, and the Middle East cultivated beans and consumed them as a staple. They paired them with a grain staple because they recognized that doing so improved the nutritional quality of both, and that the combination contained sufficient protein to sustain them. Examples of such combinations include soy and rice in China, rice and lentils in India, beans and corn in Mexico, and wheat and fava beans, chickpeas, and lentils in the Middle East. Meat and dairy were less available in these regions and so constituted a much smaller percentage of the diet. In his book *Beans Through History and Around the World*, Ken Albala asserts, ". . . without beans, the great cultures of the ancient world might never have arisen."[1] In those cultures where there was a relative scarcity of animal protein, beans occupied an important place. According to Albala, the Aztecs, Incas, and Mayas, as well as earlier cultures, made beans a central part of their diet and paired them with corn to create a nourishing source of food that led to population growth and made civilization possible.

Native Americans are said to have revered beans along with corn and squash, calling them *the three sisters* and planting them together. In Hindu and similar cultures in India, where substantial segments of the population practice vegetarianism, legumes have remained a central part of the diet for religious reasons and an important crop throughout their history.

There are also cultural reasons why people regard beans as a part of their heritage. Examples include the eating of adzuki bean paste by the Japanese, refried beans by the Mexicans, brown beans by the Swedish during certain holidays, and baked beans by Americans in the Northeastern United States, the city of Boston in particular.

Legumes were a part of the diet among the great civilizations of Egypt, Persia, and Mesopotamia. In the Old World, the cultivation of leguminous plants occupied a second, but important, place in the beginnings of agriculture, coming after grains. Remains of peas and lentils dating from 5500 B.C. have been found in Turkey. On the American continent, remains dating to 4000 B.C. demonstrate that leguminous plants appeared early in the evolution of agriculture in the

New World.

The beans that came from the New World were incorporated into the Mediterranean diet, so it is possible to say that, for centuries, dried legumes have been a basic food in the Mediterranean region, as well as in Central and South America, Mexico, the Middle East, North Africa, and China.

Dry beans are produced in pods and belong to the family of plants called legumes. The shape of the bean distinguishes it from other legumes, such as peas and lentils. Beans are usually kidney-shaped or oval, peas are round, and lentils have a flat, disklike shape. The term *dry bean* refers both to beans that are dry-packaged in sealed bags and those that are pre-cooked in cans. Dry beans include such varieties as lima, navy, pinto, and black beans, but not green beans, string beans, or soybeans.

It is basically recognized that beans are a New World crop and got distributed to Europe and Africa following Spanish and Portuguese explorations and conquests. The regions of domestication are identified as Mesoamerican, ranging from the Southern United States to Panama, with a primary focus on the Mexican, Guatemalan, and Andean regions that encompass Colombia through Peru. Mesoamerican beans are characteristically small-seeded, while Andean beans are large-seeded.

Extensive gene pools have resulted in beans of extremely diversified colors, sizes, and shapes. This diversity has been utilized in current plant-breeding programs for the development of the distinct commercial classes of beans.

They include those with:

1. A white seed coat—navy, small, white, and great Northern;

2. A solid-colored seed coat—black, kidney, small red, and pink;

3. A mottled (spotted) colored seed coat—pinto, cranberry, and yellow eye.

In researching for this book, I came across an interesting account of how legumes, also known as *pulses,* attained their nutritional prominence more than 2,000 years ago, following a ten-day experiment. In her book, *The Amazing Legume: Cooking with Lentils, Beans, & Peas*, Alice Jenner cites the author of the biblical book of Daniel (Daniel 1:12–16), as follows.[2]

Prove thy servants I beseech thee ten days and let him give us pulse to eat and water to drink, then let our countenances be looked upon before thee, and the countenances of the children that eat of the portion of the king's meat. . . . At the end of ten days their countenances appeared fatter and fairer in flesh than all the children which did eat of the portion of the king's meat. Thus Melzar took away the portion of their meat, and the wine they should drink; and gave them pulses.

This passage, whether or not you take it to heart, does reveal certain facts about legumes that cannot be disputed, even today.

1. It says that legumes are not only nutritionally comparable to meat, but are, in some respects, superior to it (they do not contain saturated fats, and they have a higher fiber content and fewer calories).

2. It lends support to the notion that legumes can fully sustain people without any ill effects if they were not to eat meat. It is also worth noting that these ancestors were favorably disposed toward scientific inquiry, even without the benefit of formal training in the scientific method.

It is not, however, my intent to advocate vegetarianism or veganism, only to make a case for increasing the consumption of legumes in the diet. From nutritional, environmental, and economic points of view, an increased consumption of legumes that ultimately leads to eating slightly less meat would be a desirable dietary change.

The populations that make legumes an integral part of their daily diet are descendants of some of the oldest inhabitants of the world. They have learned to derive most of their food from vegetable sources that were more abundant and less costly to produce. Since meat and dairy products are scarce in many parts of the world, people learned to limit their consumption of these proteins to small amounts and eat them less often. This pattern of combining larger amounts of plant-based foods with smaller portions of animal products proved to be advantageous as it protected them from an overconsumption of saturated fats and calorie-dense meats and dairy products. Plant-based foods like legumes supplied them with protein, vitamins, and minerals for nourishment, along with dietary fiber that provided bulk.

This regime, known as the Mediterranean diet, is now well-documented by epidemiologists to account for significantly lower incidences of many chronic diseases, such as heart disease, adult-onset diabetes, obesity, and certain types of cancers that plague Westerners. High intakes of the saturated fats contained in animal products, coupled with low intakes of plant-based foods, such as whole grains, vegetables, and fruits, are increasingly recognized as major factors in an unhealthy weight gain among both children and adults in Western countries, particularly the United States. An insufficient intake of plant-based foods is also depriving people of the required amount of fiber in their diets.

DRY BEANS IN EUROPEAN AND AMERICAN DIETS

Dry beans account for the greatest volume of legumes used in Europe. However, the consumption varies within individual countries and by the type of beans eaten. These differences are illustrated by a predominant use of navy beans in the United Kingdom, a preference for large white beans (great Northern, white kidney) in France, and the use of colored beans (cranberry and dark red kidney) in Italy. Western European countries (e.g. Spain, France, and the U.K.) account for about 60 percent of the total bean consumption within the European Union.

The per-capita consumption of legume-based food products in the United States, the European Union, and other industrialized economies has generally and consistently been substantially lower than that observed in other regions of the world. However, in the aggregate (with much internal variation), there has been a slight overall increase in recent years.

Total per-capita dry-bean consumption has increased gradually in the United States over the past two decades. Consumption of cooked beans is recognized as being highest in the Southern and Western areas of the country. About 55 percent of black beans, one of the fastest-growing types in terms of per-capita use, are consumed in the Southern region of the country. Although people of Hispanic origin represent approximately 11 percent of the population, they account for 33 percent of all cooked, dry, edible beans consumed. Relative to their share of the population, low-income households consume substantially more navy, lima, and pinto beans than mid- or high-income households. The popularity of such convenience items as dehydrated, extruded, frozen, and microwavable food products has led to the development of new bean products and bean formulations over the past two decades.

LEGUME CONSUMPTION IN OTHER REGIONS

The highest bean consumption in the world includes all of Latin America, where legume consumption ranges from 1 kilogram per capita per year (Argentina) to 25 kilograms per capita per year (Nicaragua). Common beans dominate and account for 87 percent of the total legume consumption in that region.

Sub-Saharan Africa utilizes a wide range of dry beans and other legume crops, such as the cowpea. These are typically cooked in water and eaten as porridge.

The subcontinent of India eats the greatest quantity and range of all the legume-based foods. They are characteristically prepared and processed in very specialized recipes.

Throughout Southeast Asia, consumption of legumes is moderate. A great variety of species are produced and used as mature seeds and immature vegetative pods. Sprouted grains are consumed fresh or dehulled, and roasted or ground for use in soups or side dishes.

Dry beans are cultivated throughout the world today. The largest commercial producers of dried common beans are Brazil, China, India, Indonesia, and the United States. This commercial production is widely distributed worldwide, with countries in Africa, Asia, Europe, Oceania, and South and North America all among the top bean growers, with Brazil and India being the largest producers.

FACTORS INFLUENCING LEGUME CONSUMPTION

The complex and long-standing differences in bean-consumption habits, which are clearly exhibited among countries, regions, or groups of people within the same country, can be explained by several factors outlined here.

Perceived Food Value

Beans are universally recognized as a wholesome and nutritious food. The traditional use of beans and maize in blended dishes is deeply embedded in Latin American cultures, for example, due in part to the fact that combining beans with the amino acids in other foods, such as grains, results in a complete protein food. Bean cultivation has been associated with having a positive impact on agriculture and the environment due to nitrogen fixation that enriches soils. This positive aspect of legumes is likely to draw more attention to its value as concerns over environmental sustainability gain momentum.

Rural vs. Urban Residence

Generally, rural populations consume greater levels of legumes than urban populations because they are more dependent on locally produced foods. It is also likely that further urbanization, with its expanded access to processed foods and increased income levels, will negatively impact bean-consumption patterns in the future.

Socioeconomic Status

People with lower incomes generally consume legumes, especially beans, more often, perpetuating the stereotypical comment that *beans are a poor man's steak*. This derogatory remark often stigmatizes the eating of beans and prevents higher utilization of them. This class distinction concerning legumes is more prevalent in the West than other regions of the world where legumes have historically and culturally enjoyed a more prominent place in everyone's diet.

Accessibility

The appreciable differences in bean costs and availability in various regions may be attributed to significant differences in global supply chains. Canned products consistently dominate bean usage in the West, compared with dry beans distributed in bulk or pre-packaged lots in other parts of the world. Canning not only adds to the cost of the product, but also contributes additives, such as salt and other preservatives, that can be unhealthy to consume on a consistent basis.

Convenience

The constraints associated with the preparation and cooking of beans and peas, such as the need for soaking, which requires advance planning, and the lengthy cooking time (raw beans and peas are not microwavable), make them less desirable for those who prefer convenience when choosing foods. This is where a case can be made for canned beans and peas; it is advisable, however, to rinse them thoroughly before consumption to remove the added salt.

Quality

Characteristic attributes that make legumes palatable, such as appearance (color, integrity), texture (firmness and consistency), taste, and flavor, are often associated with the food's quality and determine whether or not it gets chosen for consumption. In the case of beans, the additional factor of associated flatulence also plays a role in how often people want to eat them.

2

The Food Value of Legumes

Since people eat food, not nutrients, this chapter's topic refers to the food value of legumes, not their nutritional value. Even if a food is loaded with superior nutrients, if it's eaten only a little or not at all, it is of little or no value to people.

In an article titled "Why Americans Eat What They Do," authors Karen Glanz, Michael Basil, Edward Maibach, et al., examined the self-reported importance of taste, nutrition, cost, convenience, and weight control on personal dietary choices. The researchers compared study participants by age group to determine if the self-reported factors in the choice of food varied in importance among them.[1]

Cost and convenience, for example, were more important to younger people, while nutrition and weight control were more important to older persons. But taste was important to all, regarded as a minimum or standard criteria for choosing a food. Based on their findings, the authors concluded that nutritional concerns per se are of less relevance to most people than taste and cost. They suggested that nutrition-education programs should promote healthy diets as tasty and inexpensive. Of course, it would not hurt if the preparation of food was also quick, simple, and convenient for the preparer.

NUTRIENTS CONTRIBUTED BY LEGUMES
TO RECOMMENDED DAILY VALUES IN DIET

Based on a 2,000-calorie diet, a half-cup serving of legumes contains, on average, the following nutrients in the proportions of their recommended daily values (DV):

- 50 percent of folic acid (a B vitamin);

- 50 percent of manganese;

- 25 percent of fiber;

- 10 percent each of copper, iron, magnesium, potassium, and protein;

- 6–8 percent of selenium and zinc.

The third item in this list, fiber, also called roughage, is not a nutrient, but an indigestible carbohydrate from plants. There are two types of fiber, soluble and insoluble, and both provide different benefits to the body.

Soluble fiber acts like a scavenger by binding with, and removing, cholesterol from the body, thereby reducing the cholesterol level.

Insoluble fiber, consisting mostly of cellulose, acts as bulk and slows the emptying of the stomach, keeping you satisfied for a longer period of time. This slowing also maintains a steady level of blood sugar and prevents sudden spikes and dips. In addition, the bulk aids in moving the contents of the large intestine, keeping you regular.

The folic acid in legumes plays a key role in averting heart disease by keeping the blood levels of homocysteine low. A high level of homocysteine is associated with an increased risk of developing atherosclerosis or hardening of arteries.

The protein in legumes is plant-based and does not contain cholesterol or saturated fats, only a small amount of polyunsaturated fat. Unlike the protein in animal-based sources, such as meats and dairy, the protein in legumes is lean. A serving of legumes also contains a generous dose of flavonoids, the heart-healthy phytochemicals (researchers say as much as in a glass of red wine). In an article titled "Loving Legumes for All the Right Reasons: Health, Flavor and Value," author

Sharon Palmer declares legumes—beans, peas, and lentils—to be as close to a perfect food as you can find. She explains her assertion in terms of the significant contribution a single one-half cup of legumes makes to the recommended daily values (DV).[2]

Is there any nutrient lacking in legumes? Yes, there is one essential amino acid called methionine that, with the exception of soybeans, is not present in legumes in sufficient quantity to meet the body's daily requirement. Proteins are made up of twenty different amino acids in various sequences. Nearly half of them are made or recycled by the body, but the remaining essential amino acids must be obtained through the daily diet. Adult humans need nine of these—histdine, isoleucine, leucine, lycine, methionine, phenylalanine, threonine, tryptophan, and valine. Infants and young children also need a tenth amino acid, arginine, from food. A food that contains all the essential amino acids in sufficient quantities to meet the daily requirement is considered a complete protein source, and a food that is missing one or more of the essential amino acids in sufficient quantities is regarded as an incomplete protein source. Eating a complementary food, such as corn or rice, easily makes up the missing amino acid in legumes. It is not necessary to eat the two foods in the same meal as long as both are included in meals eaten during the course of the day. This is something our ancestors seem to have gleaned intuitively as they always combined legumes with corn, maize, or rice.

The nutritional advantage of legumes seems truly magnified when you take into account the nutritional content of its animal-food counterpart. A 5-ounce steak (average serving size), for example, contains 300 calories, 44 grams of protein, 120 milligrams of cholesterol, 12 grams of fat (most of it saturated), and zero fiber. One half a cup of lentils, on the other hand, contains 115 calories, 8.9 grams of protein, no cholesterol, 1.3 grams of fat, all of it polyunsaturated, and 7.8 grams of fiber. Yet, lentils literally cost pennies per serving while the steak can run into several dollars. Although it's not my intent to advocate total abstinence from meat eating, I do believe that a reduction in meat consumption, especially red meat, along with eating more legumes would go a long way toward lowering the health risks associated with eating calorie-dense foods containing saturated fats, cholesterol, and little or no fiber. A half-cup serving of legumes daily is consistent with the *Dietary Guidelines for Americans,* developed by the U.S. Department of Health and Human Services (USDHHS) and the U.S. Department of Agriculture (USDA), that recommend 3 cups of legumes per week.[3]

HEALTH BENEFITS OF EATING LEGUMES

Legumes are considered super foods, and by definition a super food has to do more than simply nourish and provide energy. It has to have significant additional benefits for overall health and well-being. Drawing from the fact that many ancient civilizations not only sustained themselves on plant-based legumes and grains, but generally lived free of today's many diseases and health problems, researchers have sought to find out if legume consumption could be associated with lower rates of certain diseases, heart disease, and certain types of cancer in particular. The results of their efforts have not been disappointing. There is ever-increasing scientific evidence pointing to the positive health benefits of diets high in whole grains, legumes, fruits, vegetables, nuts, fish, low-fat dairy products, and less meat (red and processed meat in particular). This may sound like the Mediterranean diet, because the principal components are akin to it. The major benefits of such a diet are derived from lean protein, fiber, and the low amounts of polyunsaturated fats from legumes and grains combined with lower amounts of saturated fats and minerals, such as iron from meats and dairy products.

Currently, there's a mountain of evidence-based data showing that if red meat, along with its processed varieties like bacon and salami, is consumed regularly, the risk of dying from such diseases as heart disease, diabetes, and some cancers is increased. A recent major diet and health study, conducted by the National Institutes of Health (NIH) and the American Association of Retired Persons (AARP) in 2009 revealed just that.[4]

More than 50,000 men and women participated in this study, which examined how meat consumption affects mortality over a ten-year period. The intake of three categories of meats—red meat (beef and pork), white meat (poultry and fish), and processed meat (bacon, sausage, lunch meats, cold cuts, ham, and hot dogs) was examined. Those who ate the most red meat had a 31-percent higher death rate than those who ate the least. A 16-percent higher death rate was associated with processed-meat consumption. The study's findings held up even after other health habits and risk factors were taken into account. Cardiovascular and cancer mortalities followed the same pattern as total mortality in this study.

Drawing from the findings of this and other research, Harvey Simon of Harvard Medical School pointed to a link between red-meat consumption and increased risk for premature death, heart disease, colon cancer, and other malignancies in a two-part article entitled "Meat or Beans: What Will You Have?" As healthier alternatives to red and processed meats, Simon recommended fish, poultry, and legumes as excellent choices.[5,6]

Given the impressive array of antioxidant and anti-inflammatory phytonutrients in legumes, it is not surprising that numerous studies have connected legume intake with a reduced risk for certain cancers, especially colon cancer. Chronic excessive oxidative stress and chronic inflammation are both risk factors for the development of many types of cancer. By increasing the body's supply of antioxidant and anti-inflammatory nutrients, legumes can help lower the cancer risk. Although most of the studies linking legume intake with disease risk have been done on laboratory animals, they have been largely consistent in their findings.

The implicit message in the research findings on the diet/disease connection is not total abstinence from meats—even the researchers who conducted the studies do not advocate this. Instead, it is to cut down on portions of meats, especially red meats, eat them less often, and include more plant-based foods, such as legumes, in the daily diet.

❧ 3 ❧

Straight Talk on Buzzwords

Everyone has heard or used one or more of the following buzz-words in conversations, or has come across them in reading. The words are, however, sometimes used without a full awareness of what they mean in relation to how our bodies function, or if the underlying concept points to a benefit or a harm for the body.

■ ANTIOXIDANTS

Oxidation, one of the body's natural chemical processes, can produce free radicals, which are highly unstable molecules known to cause damage to cells, and this cell damage is known to play a role in heart disease and cancer, among other conditions. Free radicals are produced, for example, when the body breaks down food that is to be used for energy or storage. They are also released when the body is exposed to chemicals, radiation, and environmental contaminants. The balance between the free radicals generated and the antioxidants the body produces as natural defense mechanisms determines the extent of the cell damage. Foods or supplements containing antioxidants boost the body's defense against free radicals and counter the oxidative stress and associated cell damage. Antioxidants are found in many foods, such as brightly colored fruits and vegetables, grains, nuts, meats, poultry, and fish. Some known antioxidant powerhouses include berries (most), broccoli, cantaloupes, carrots, collard greens, fish and shellfish, green peppers, kale, soybeans, squash, sweet potatoes, tomatoes, and red wine.

■ BODY MASS INDEX (BMI)

Body mass index (BMI) is a number calculated by using a formula that takes a person's height and weight into consideration. The BMI does not measure body fat directly, but research has shown that it correlates to direct measures of body fat, such as underwater weighing. The index provides a reliable indicator of body fat for most people and is used to screen for weight categories that may lead to health problems. However, a BMI is not a diagnostic tool, and a healthcare provider would need to perform further assessments to determine if excess weight is a health risk. Such assessments might include evaluations of diet, physical activity, family history, and other appropriate health screenings.

If using the metric system, the formula is weight in kilograms divided by height in meters squared. Example: height = 1.65 meters; weight = 68 kg, BMI = 68/2.7225 or 24.98. If the formula uses weight in pounds, they are divided by height in inches squared and multiplied by a conversion factor of 703. Example: weight = 150 lbs; height = 65", BMI = [150/(65 x 65)] x 703 = 24.96. The values in both examples can be rounded to 25.0. BMI tables are widely available, including from your healthcare provider, and they can provide easy reference without having to calculate it yourself. You can check your BMI for your particular height and weight and find out if you fall within the normal, overweight, or obese categories. According to the BMI weight-status categories, anyone with a BMI over 25 would be classified as overweight and anyone with a BMI over 30 would be classified as obese. Although the BMI number is calculated the same way for children and adults of either gender, the criteria used to interpret the meaning of the BMI number for children and teens differ from those used for adults.

■ CHOLESTEROL

Cholesterol is a necessary fatlike substance present in the cell membranes of all higher animals. It is a precursor of bile acids and steroid hormones. The liver and other tissues synthesize most of the cholesterol, but some is absorbed from foods of animal origin in our diet. Plant-based foods do not contain cholesterol. It is carried in the plasma by specific lipoproteins (fats attached to proteins). There are two major types of cholesterol circulating in the blood, the high-density lipoprotein (HDL), the good cholesterol; and the low-density lipoprotein (LDL), the bad cholesterol. The amount of protein coating—the waxy, fatlike substance—determines the density of the lipoprotein. An abnormally high level of LDL cholesterol is often associated with atherosclerosis, or hardening of the arteries. HDL, on the other hand, promotes the transport of cholesterol to the liver for excretion in the bile. Normal adult levels of blood cholesterol are 150–200 mg/dl. Cholesterol in itself is not believed to be the culprit for heart disease. It is the inflammation of the blood vessels that creates the problem. Since only foods of animal origin contain cholesterol, it is advisable to limit their intake and add more plant-based foods to the diet. Plant-based foods, legumes for example, have the added benefit of being high in both soluble and insoluble fiber. The soluble fiber binds itself to fatty acids in the blood and, acting as a scavenger, removes them from the body.

■ ESSENTIAL AMINO ACIDS

Proteins are made up of amino acids, which are regarded as the building blocks of the human body. They are a part of every cell, tissue, and organ in the body, and are essential for many bodily functions, such as building and repairing tissue, and making enzymes, hormones, and biochemicals. There are twenty different amino acids that join together to make protein. While the body makes a majority of the amino acids in the required proportions, there are eight amino acids (nine in children) that the body does not make in the amount needed by the human body. These are known as essential amino acids, because it is essential that you get them through the food you eat. The protein sources in the diet are labeled according to how many of the essential amino acids they provide in sufficient amount needed by the body. A complete protein source is one that provides all of the essential amino acids. Animal-based foods, including dairy products, eggs, poultry, and seafood, are considered complete protein sources. Soybean and soybean products, such as tofu, are the only plant-based foods that provide all eight essential amino acids, and they are considered a source of complete protein. An incomplete protein source is one that is low in one or more of the essential amino acids. Complementary proteins are two or more incomplete protein sources that together provide adequate amounts of all the essential amino acids. Legumes are an example of an incomplete protein because they lack one of the essential amino acids, methionine, in the quantity sufficient for the human body. When combined with a complimentary grain (rice or corn, for example) that provides the missing essential amino acid, legumes provide the body with all the essential amino acids it requires.

■ FIBER

Dietary fiber, also known as roughage or bulk, is found mainly in fruits, legumes, vegetables, and whole grains. Unlike other food components, such as fats, proteins, or carbohydrates, which are broken down and absorbed, fiber is a part of plant foods that the body cannot digest or absorb. Fiber, therefore, passes relatively intact through the stomach, small intestine, and colon and is excreted out of the body. In the process, however, it performs several important functions in maintaining not only digestive health, but also overall health.

There are two types of dietary fiber, one, insoluble fiber, that does not dissolve in water, and two, soluble fiber, that does dissolve in water, and each serves a different, useful function. The amount of each type of fiber varies in different plant foods, and eating a wide variety of plant-based foods ensures enough of both kinds to derive maximum health benefits.

Soluble fiber converts into a gel-like substance in the digestive tract, and acts as a scavenger for bad cholesterol. It binds itself to particles of LDL (the bad cholesterol) in the small intestine and prevents them from entering the bloodstream, thereby lowering the level of circulating LDL. Soluble fiber also helps control blood-sugar levels by slowing the absorption of any sugar in the food, and preventing the sudden rise and fall of glucose levels in the blood. This is particularly beneficial to people with adult-onset diabetes. Soluble fiber is found in apples, barley, beans, carrots, lentils, oat bran, oranges and other citrus fruits, and peas.

Insoluble fiber increases stool bulk and helps keep people regular. High-fiber foods are believed to help in preventing weight gain by taking longer to empty out of the stomach, which leads to feeling full for longer periods, thereby keeping hunger at bay. They also tend to contain fewer calories for the same volume of food than such low-fiber foods as meats. Fruits, nuts, vegetables, and wheat bran, are all good sources of insoluble fiber.

■ FLAVONOIDS

Flavonoids are plant-based compounds with powerful antioxidant properties. They help reduce inflammation in the body, promote healthy arteries, and help fight aging by preventing and repairing cellular damage. Flavonoids are being increasingly studied for their properties that protect against dementia, Alzheimer's disease, and some cancers. As many as 4,000 flavonoids have been identified thus far, and many of them are found in everyday foods and beverages. Eating a diverse diet that regularly includes such foods as apples (the flavonoids are in the skin), blueberries, broccoli, cabbage, capers, dark chocolate, onions, red grapes, red wine, strawberries, and tea (all kinds) will provide an adequate daily dose of flavonoids. Oh yes, add beer to this list too—the antioxidant property of the flavonoids found in beer is believed to exceed that of red wine, soy, and tea.

■ GLYCEMIC INDEX

All orally consumed foods and drinks trigger a metabolic response from the body. As food gets processed, the body does one of two things with the product— stores it in the tissue as fat, or burns it as energy. Humans are genetically hardwired to shunt foods into fat cells whenever possible, as that ensures survival. Whether food is stored or immediately utilized as energy depends on the glycemic index (GI) and the glycemic load (GL) of the food item. Foods have been assigned a glycemic index number based on the comparative increases in blood-sugar levels they produce when that food is consumed.

All foods and drinks can be categorized as either high or low glycemic. A low-glycemic food causes a slower and more gradual rise in blood sugar than a high-glycemic food. If the food item has a high GI and GL, it will be stored primarily as fat, and if it has a low GI and GL, it will primarily be used for energy. Quickly digested and metabolized foods possess the highest glycemic indices, which means they elevate blood glucose and insulin levels and cause fat storage. These high-glycemic foods increase blood-sugar concentration quickly, leading to insulin release in response, which, in turn, brings the blood sugar down rapidly, triggering hunger. Low-glycemic foods, on the other hand, are digested slowly, keeping you feeling full longer. Because they release glucose into the bloodstream gradually, with a corresponding slow release of insulin, they do not trigger rapid hunger.

Another way of interpreting the glycemic index is to think of it as a measure of how fast, and by how much, a food raises blood-sugar levels. Examples of high-GI foods include concentrated sugary foods, such as doughnuts and ice cream, white rice, and white bread. Examples of low-GI foods include brown rice, legumes, quinoa, and whole-grain bread.

■ MACRONUTRIENTS

Macronutrients are those compounds in food—carbohydrates, proteins, and fats—that are essential to sustain life. The general rule of thumb in dietary guidelines is that 55 percent of the body's requirements for nourishment must be obtained from carbohydrates (grains, pasta, potatoes, sugary drinks, sweets), 30 percent from fats (oils, dairy products, nuts), and 15 percent from proteins (meat, poultry, fish, legumes).

■ MICRONUTRIENTS

There are two categories of micronutrients—vitamins and minerals—that contain the chemical compounds needed to carry on many bodily functions. Each micronutrient aids in specific functions. Vitamin A is important for good eyesight, appropriate immune function, and the growth of tissues. The vitamin-B group is essential to energy metabolism, blood-cell development, and maintaining the health of the nervous system. Calcium keeps the bones strong and can help prevent osteoporosis. Iron is necessary in the production of hemoglobin in blood. A well-balanced diet containing the recommended servings of fruits and vegetables generally ensures that the body gets the required amounts of the essential vitamins and minerals. However, during periods of additional demands on the body, such as during pregnancy, additional amounts, in the form of dietary supplements, are recommended.

■ METABOLISM

The term applies to the sum of the physical and chemical processes in the body that convert food into fuel and make it available to use as needed. The body's fuel needs vary, depending on such factors as age, gender, weight, and physical activity. The minimum amount required by a person to perform normal body functions at rest, including breathing, digestion, and maintaining a normal heart rate, is measured in terms of calories or kilocalories and is referred to as the basal metabolic rate (BMR). Stated another way, the BMR is the rate at which the body uses fuel while at rest to keep vital functions going. It is possible to calculate how many calories you need in the course of the day. For example, a forty-year-old man who weighs 200 pounds and does hard physical labor requires 3,370 calories per day to maintain his weight. A forty-year-old woman who weighs 140 pounds and engages in moderate physical activity needs only 2,150 calories per day to maintain her weight.

Not everyone burns calories at the same rate. An overweight person uses more calories than a normal weight person just to sustain him or herself. This is the reason why even a small reduction in calorie intake at the start of dieting results in a significant weight loss. A weight loss is generally followed by a lower BMR, which makes it increasingly harder to lose weight if no further reduction is made in calorie intake. A drastic reduction in calorie intake, however, can be harmful to health and should be done only under the supervision of a healthcare provider.

■ OMEGA-3 FATTY ACIDS

Often simply referred to as omega-3s, these are polyunsaturated essential fatty acids needed by the body for normal functioning. Since they are not made by the body, they need to be obtained from the diet. There are several types of omega-3 fatty acids, but the two most important ones are EPA and DHA. Both are found primarily in fish and algae, although flaxseeds and some other plant foods contain the precursor to them known as ALA. Omega-3s are known to play a key role in reducing inflammation in the body that is associated with many cardiovascular diseases, such as heart disease, high blood pressure, and stroke. For this reason, the omega-3s are considered heart healthy, and are one of the reasons behind the dietary recommendation to eat fish at least 1–2 times a week. Coldwater fish, such as black cod, bluefish, herring, mackerel, salmon, and sardines, are especially rich sources of omega-3s. According to the 2010 *Dietary Guidelines for Americans,* recommendations for a daily intake of omega-3s are 0.7–1.6 grams per day, depending on age and gender.

■ OMEGA-6 FATTY ACIDS

Omega-6s are also essential polyunsaturated fatty acids like the omega-3s, which the body does not make, and must also be provided through the diet. They are found in eggs, meats, nuts, poultry, seeds, including legumes, and vegetable oils (corn, peanut, safflower, soybean, and sunflower). Linoleic acid, or LA, and gamma-linoleic acid, or GLA, are two types of unsaturated omega-6 fatty acids. Recommendations for a daily intake of omega-6s are 7–16 grams per day, depending on age and gender. People in North America typically consume 11–30 times more omega-6 fatty acids in their diet than omega-3 fatty acids. Some experts believe this imbalance in favor of omega-6s is contributing to the rising rate of inflammatory disorders, such as arthritis, cancer, and coronary heart disease, in the United States. Since the two fats work in different ways to protect health, a more balanced proportion of omega-3s and omega-6s in the diet, or through dietary supplements, is highly beneficial.

■ PHYTOCHEMICALS

Phytochemicals are plant chemicals that have protective or disease-preventing properties. Plants produce these chemicals to protect themselves, and research has shown they also protect humans against some types of cancer and other diseases. Specifically, it has been shown that certain phytochemicals help prevent the formation of potential carcinogens and/or act on cells to suppress cancer development.

Many different types of phytochemicals are found in fruits and vegetables, grains, legumes, and nuts. Examples include lycopene in tomatoes, isoflavones in soybean, and flavonoids in fruits and vegetables—apples, blueberries, cherries, cranberries, broccoli, cabbage, carrots, and cauliflower—as well as in tea. Regular consumption of fruits and vegetables, grains, legumes, and nuts provides sufficient phytochemicals to protect against disease. At present, there is no scientific evidence to support taking phytochemical supplements, but studies are ongoing.

■ SATURATED FATS

These are fats in which the carbon atoms are saturated with hydrogen atoms and are solid at room temperature. The solid fat that is floating on top in refrigerated leftover stew, or in an open can of meat stew is typically a saturated fat. Fats from animal foods—meats, poultry, whole-fat milk, yogurt, ice cream, butter, and cheese—are primary sources of saturated fat in the diet, but there are also plant oils, such as coconut oils, palm oils, vegetable shortening, and cocoa butter, that are sources of saturated fats. These latter plant oils are often added to commercially prepared baked goods, such as cakes, cookies, doughnuts, and pies. Saturated fat raises LDL, the bad cholesterol, and for that reason warrants a limit on its intake. Higher levels of LDL can increase your risk for heart disease and adult-onset diabetes.

In a well-balanced diet, 25–35 percent of your total daily calories can come from fat, but saturated fat should contribute no more than 10 percent (some experts recommend lowering it to 7 percent) of total daily calories. When buying pre-packaged foods, it is important to read the nutrition label for the amount of saturated fat (in grams) per serving and figure out what percentage of calories it is contributing to your diet.

Some effective ways to limit saturated fat in your diet are:

- To avoid marbled meats that have fat embedded in them, choosing instead lean cuts of meat or those with visible fat that can be trimmed;

- To remove skin from chicken and other poultry before cooking;

- To use low-fat spreads instead of butter; and

- To substitute high-fat desserts with low- or reduced-fat versions that contain significantly less saturated fat.

■ MONOUNSATURATED FAT

This is a type of unsaturated fat found in a variety of foods and oils that remains liquid at room temperature. Sources of monounsaturated fats are avocados, nuts, and vegetable oils (canola, olive, safflower, and sunflower). Studies show that eating foods rich in monounsaturated fat improves blood cholesterol levels, thereby helping to decrease the risk for heart disease, and maintains balanced blood-sugar levels, which can keep adult-onset diabetes under control.

■ POLYUNSATURATED FAT

Polyunsaturated fat is a type of unsaturated fat, found mostly in seafood and some plant-based foods and oils, that remains liquid at room temperature. The often-touted omega-3s and omega-6s are types of polyunsaturated fats, and both are credited as being heart healthy. When consumed regularly, the polyunsaturated fats found in certain fish in abundance—particularly salmon, trout, and herring—as well as in canola oil, soybean oil, walnuts, and flaxseed, are known to lower the risk of coronary artery disease. These fats are also credited with protecting against irregular heartbeat, and helping to lower blood pressure.

■ TRANS FATS

Also referred to as trans-fatty acid (TFA), trans fat is formed when hydrogen is added to liquid vegetable oils to convert them into a solid fat through a process called hydrogenation. More than other types of fat, trans fats are known to raise the LDL, the bad cholesterol level, and lower the level of HDL, the good cholesterol, both of which increase the risk for heart disease. For this reason, trans fats are regarded as doubly unhealthy. Scientists are not sure why hydrogenation has this effect, but one theory is that adding hydrogen to oil makes the oil more difficult to digest.

Trans fat also has other harmful effects, such as causing a rise in triglycerides, a type of fat found in blood that is known to contribute to the hardening of the arteries—atherosclerosis—and inflammation in the body, both causing blockage in the blood vessels of the heart. Trans fat is used in manufacturing foods, to keep them fresh longer and feeling less greasy, with a longer shelf life. It is found in shortening used in cooking, some margarines, and in processed foods like baked goods, cakes, crackers, and other snack foods. The American Heart Association recommends that people consume no more than 2 grams of trans fat per day. However the Food and Drug Administration guidelines allow manufacturers of any food product with less than 0.5 grams of trans fat to list it as containing 0 grams on the nutrition label. But there is another way to tell if trans fats are present in a food. If the ingredients listed on a packaged food label contain the words *hydrogenated* or *partially hydrogenated* oils or shortening, know that the food contains trans fat, and limit its intake.

❦ 4 ❦

Health Implications of Changes in the Traditional Diet of Selected Countries

Before the development of agriculture and animal husbandry, dietary choices for humans would have been necessarily limited to unprocessed or minimally processed wild plant and animal foods. With the initial domestication of plants and animals, the nutrient characteristics of these formerly wild foods changed, slowly and subtly at first, but more rapidly with the advancing technology that followed the industrial revolution.

The advent of agriculture also introduced novel foods as staples for which the human genome had little evolutionary experience. More importantly, after the industrial revolution, previously unknown food-processing procedures and combinations were developed. These novel foods—cereals, dairy products, refined sugars and vegetable oils, and alcohol—that make up a significant proportion of today's diet would not have been a part of the typical pre-industrial or pre-agricultural-era diet. Refined sugar is a prime example of a food with no precedent during human evolution that is now consumed in increasing quantities. The first evidence of crystalline-sucrose production appears about 500 BC in Northern India. Before this time, honey would have represented one of the few concentrated sugars to which people would have had access. The consumption of refined sugar has further changed with the advent of technology in the late 1970s that made it economically feasible to manufacture high-fructose corn syrup

(HFCS) in mass quantity and replace the more expensive sugar in food processing. The digestion, absorption, and metabolism of fructose differs from that of glucose, and dietary fructose may well be responsible for an increased weight gain, as the use of HFCS in the United States has mirrored the rapid rise in the rates of overweight and obesity.[1]

Regular consumption of increasingly larger portions of food, coupled with changes in lifestyle have given rise to what is referred to as the *diseases of civilization* that include heart disease, cancer, and adult-onset diabetes. Virtually all of these diseases are caused by complex dietary elements, as well as environmental and genetic factors. Coronary heart disease, for example, does not arise simply from excessive saturated fat in the diet, but rather from a complex interaction of nutritional factors directly linked to the consumption of newly developed foods. These foods, in turn, adversely influence biochemical processes in the body, leading to, or exacerbating, chronic diseases. The ultimate cause underlying diseases of civilization is believed to be the collision of our ancient genetic makeup with the new conditions of life in affluent nations, including the nutritional elements of recently introduced foods.

In the United States and most other Western countries, diet-related chronic diseases represent the single largest cause of morbidity and mortality. These diseases are epidemic in contemporary Westernized people and typically affect 50–65 percent of the adults. Yet these were rare or nonexistent in hunter-gatherers, and are far less prevalent in today's non-Western populations, although a growing number of them are gradually adopting Western-type diets. To date, Western experience has demonstrated that such a shift will likely lead to an increase in diet-related diseases, which would add to the existing burden of other communicable diseases that are still prevalent in those countries. The rising prevalence of these diet-related diseases exacts a high cost on societies everywhere, both in terms of the health and welfare of individuals and the pressure on the national health systems, and it is creating an urgent need to find solutions to this burgeoning problem. This has prompted epidemiologists, public-health scientists who study distribution and determinants of health and disease around the world, to gather data on diet-related chronic diseases over the past several decades. Their efforts have shed some light on dietary trends and patterns, and their corresponding effect on chronic diseases.[2,3,4]

In the last decades of the twentieth century, massive amounts of data were being collected, compiled, and published in the United States about the diet/disease connection, especially as it related to chronic diseases. The data pointed to dietary fat, especially saturated fat, as the main culprit, and this led to recommendations for a reduction in dietary-fat intake, and an increase in the consumption of vegetables, fruits, and cereal grains. There were no consistent or specific recommendations for achieving a significantly reduced intake of dietary fat, and many, including the National Academy of Sciences Committee on Diet, Nutrition, and Cancer, viewed a reduced-fat intake to 30 percent of total calories as inadequate—the Academy took the position that the available data justified an even greater reduction.

Overall, a broader understanding about the diet/disease connection needs to be gained by looking at not only the national experience, but also the experience of people around the world.

■ EVOLUTION OF THE DIET IN MEDITERRANEAN COUNTRIES

The Mediterranean diet is long believed to hold promise for mitigating the adverse effects of Western dietary patterns. The traditional Mediterranean diet is characterized by a high intake of vegetables, legumes, fruits, nuts, cereals (largely unrefined in the past), and olive oil, coupled with a low intake of saturated fats, such as those present in meats and poultry. Frequent, moderately high intake of fish, low-to-moderate intake of dairy products, and regular but moderate consumption of alcohol, mainly in the form of wine drunk during meals, are also a part of this diet. Interest in the Mediterranean diet was sparked with the work of Ancel Keys in the 1950s when he and some colleagues studied the risks for coronary heart disease in seven countries and found links from high-fat diets to higher concentrations of blood cholesterol and a higher risk of heart disease.[4]

During the early 1960s, people living in the Mediterranean region enjoyed some of the highest life expectancies and lowest rates of coronary heart disease. Since these favorable health statistics were not attributable to economic status, education level, or healthcare expenditure, researchers began to focus on the region's diet. As a result, they gained some insights into how the Mediterranean diet has been faring in the Mediterranean region itself, taking into account the socio-economic transformations and related diet transitions of the last few decades.

Greece

Pooling data from a number of well-designed national surveys, the National Statistical Service of Greece examined the dietary consumption patterns in Greece during the period 1957 to 2005.[5] This data that spanned nearly half a century revealed many significant trends, and patterns about the Greek diet.

First, in the post–World War II period there were drastic changes in dietary patterns among the Greeks. The Mediterranean diet, an established, centuries-old tradition, mainly consisting of cereal (bread), vegetables, legumes, fruits, olive oil, wine, lamb, and goat meat, has been gradually declining, and even disappearing, in Greece. It was observed that there was a gradual reduction in consumers' demand for their traditional foods up to the year 1974, and this was accompanied by a rise in the consumption of a Western-style diet that included an increasing use of processed foods, convenience foods, and more and different animal foods. Added to this, a large increase in meat consumption in the Greek diet was recorded in the Household Budget Survey of 1974, and continued until the end of the 1990s.

In the 1980s in Greece, another new trend of eating meals not prepared at home emerged, and that led to a progressive increase in food expenditure away from home. This trend took root and led to today's dietary habits in Greece of eating more Western-European and North-American types of meats and less fresh vegetables, potatoes, and especially legumes, whose intake was cut in half. This is noteworthy, given the importance of legumes as an integral part of the traditional Greek diet, reflected in the bean soup being regarded as the national dish.

Following this dietary transformation, Greece has, not surprisingly, emerged as having the highest rate of obesity (body mass index of 30 and over) in Europe and the world. In the early 2000s, the International Obesity Task Force, working in collaboration with the European Association for the Study of Obesity, placed Greece at the top in the ranks of obesity in Europe.[6] The Greek population had lost the premium position it held (next to the Japanese) in life expectancy at a global level until the 1970s. Greek men fell to the twelfth position, with 77.2 years, while Greek women slipped down to eighteenth place in life expectancy in the '90s from the sixth place that they had held in the 1970s. In 2006, with an average age of 79.5 years, Swedish men were found to have the longest life expectancy at a pan-European level.

The shift from traditional to Western-European and North-American type diet does not bode well for the traditional Mediterranean diet, which seems to be on the decline even in Greece and Crete, its presumed birthplace. Except for the continued high consumption of olive oil and fresh fruits and vegetables in Greece, more recent food-consumption patterns there have moved away from those close to the Mediterranean diet that were prevalent as recently as the mid 1960s. Shifts that accompanied rapid urbanization, growing incomes, technical changes in the food industry, rapid expansion of fast-food outlets, and globalization have led to the greatly increased consumption of animal products, fats other than olive oil, and sugar.

In the mid 1960s, the average national food consumption in Greece was 2,900 kilocalories per person per day, with 29 percent coming from fats (13 percent of it from olive oil) and 43 percent from cereals. Meat consumption was a mere 33 kilograms per person per year, and sugar was 18 kilograms (raw sugar equivalent). Three and a half decades later, the consumption had risen to 3,700 kilocalories per day per person, with fats accounting for 36 percent of the total calories (12 percent from olive oil), meat consumption doubling to 88 kilograms and sugar consumption rising to 32 kilograms per person per year.[7]

In a study conducted jointly by the University of Athens Medical School and the Harvard School of Public Health, researchers sought to answer the question "Does adherence to a Mediterranean diet improve total mortality, as well as mortality due to coronary heart disease and cancer?" They used the data from the Greek component of the European Prospective Investigation of Cancer and Nutrition (EPIC) study that took place between 1994 and 1999. From all regions of Greece, a total of 28,572 men and women between the ages of twenty and eighty-six participated in this study. Baseline measurements of diet were obtained using a food-frequency questionnaire. Adherence to the traditional Mediterranean diet (incorporating nine prominent components of it) was determined using a ten-point scale from zero to nine, with higher scores indicating greater adherence to the diet. The results, published in *The New England Journal of Medicine,* revealed some striking findings about the association between the degree of adherence to a traditional Mediterranean diet and overall mortality, as well as mortality due to coronary heart disease (CHD) and cancer in the Greek population.[8]

Adherence to the traditional Mediterranean diet was inversely related to overall mortality. Even a modest two-point increase in the aggregate score in adherence to the diet was associated with a significant reduction of overall mortality, as well as deaths from cardiovascular disease and cancer. In the fields of medicine and public health, this phenomenon is referred to as the *dose response,* meaning the higher the dose of the cause (a certain type of diet in this case), the higher the effect, positive or negative. Based on their findings, the researchers concluded that adherence to the Mediterranean diet is associated with a significant reduction in total mortality as well as coronary heart and cancer mortality. Individual components of the diet were found not to be generally predictive of total mortality, suggesting that multiple dietary components are necessary to yield the most protective effect.

Spain

Spain, a fairly new member of the European Union, has a somewhat different experience than Greece with respect to its dietary transition. It is a country that modernized later than most European countries. During the latter part of the twentieth century, Spain experienced rapid economic change, with the past thirty to forty years showing important socioeconomic, and consequently food-behavior modifications. In 1950, the Spanish population was half urban, and by 1995, it was three-quarters urban. The occupational structure of Spain around this time began to resemble that of other Western European countries, and was associated with a major reduction in demands for physical labor at work. Spain has since exhibited some new trends, such as a high-fat diet, high obesity levels, and associated health problems that had not been prevalent before

Spanish dietary data is gathered through a series of nationally representative household budget surveys and is available for three different time periods—1964–1965, 1980–1981, and 1990–1991. The food-intake data was collected from more than 20,000 households in the course of a full week. The trends revealed that the Spanish diet contained very high levels of fat, increased amounts of meat, a greatly increased intake of dairy, plus a high-fruit and low-vegetable intake. The proportion of plant-based foods eaten decreased significantly during the same period.

Consumption of cereals, grain products, legumes, and potatoes were all reduced to half their 1964–1965 levels. Vegetable intake increased slightly during this period, but the major positive shift was a two-fold increase in fruit consumption. The amount of dairy and fruit consumed in Spain is among the highest in Europe, far above the other Mediterranean countries. Also, the high consumption of monounsaturated fat and the high combined ratio of mono- and polyunsaturated fats (like olive oil) to saturated fats provide an important dimension to the Spanish diet. While wine consumption in Spain decreased continuously from 1961 to 1993 and hard-liquor consumption remained stable, the consumption of beer increased during this period.[9]

High rates of obesity and adult overweight are quite prevalent in Spain, particularly among men and are second only to Greece. The researchers contend that the overweight problem may be stemming partly from the diet and partly from reduced physical activity as the result of a shift towards sedentary work, with less leisure time spent in physical activity. Furthermore, the authors suggest that weight control and physical fitness are not as important in Spain as elsewhere in the European Union. Interestingly, however, the rates of cardiovascular diseases and cancer mortality are lower than you would expect in a population with a high obesity rate. It is believed that the harmful effects of the high-fat intake are offset by the high proportional intake of the combined mono-and poly-unsaturated fat to saturated fat. The leading causes of death in Spain since 1980 have been due to diseases of the circulatory system, followed by cancer. After 1980, in a trend seen throughout Europe, there has been a decrease in mortality from diseases of the circulatory system, but an increase in deaths from cancer in Spain.

The transition in Spanish nutrition, with its increase in both dietary fat and fruit intake, markedly correlates with the decrease in mortality from diseases of the circulatory system. The increase in dietary fat is primarily due to a sharp increase in the consumption of meat and dairy products, both of which contribute to a rise in the level of cholesterol. Given the long-held association between high serum cholesterol level and cardiovascular disease, the unexpected diminishing of cardiovascular mortality has been called the *Spanish Paradox,* and can possibly be explained by the interacting of many cardiovascular risk and protective factors. Figuring prominently in the protective category are the antioxidants and phytochemicals derived from plant-based foods like fruits and vegetables. The consumption of fruits in Spain is the highest in Europe. Greece is the other European Mediterranean country with a high-fruit intake and a high total fruit-and-vegetable intake, and that country is experiencing an *increase* in cardiovascular mortality, the opposite of the trend in Spain. The lower cardiovascular mortality in Spain is explained, at least in part, by improved medical care there.

Italy

The United States Center for Nutrition Policy and Promotion, in collaboration with the University of North Carolina, looked at the dietary trends and patterns in the United States and Italy for the period 1961–1992. The purpose of the investigation was to find out if the idealized traditional Mediterranean diet still existed in Italy, then compare what they found with the prevailing U.S. diet, and ultimately determine the feasibility of introducing the Mediterranean diet as a model for eating habits in the United States.

They examined the U.S. and Italian food data, regarded the best available source of information for both countries at the time. During the thirty-year period of the study, per-capita food consumption increased in both the U.S. and Italy, and in both countries they found considerably reduced intakes in whole milk and white potatoes. In the United States they found less consumption of eggs and red meat, and in Italy, they found a lower intake of grains. In Italy, however, the use of milk from such animals as goats, ewes, and buffaloes (but not cows), was more typical, especially for making cheese. In the United States, the use of low-fat milk steadily increased, reaching a level by 1986 that was four times higher than its use in Italy. Even with the reduced intake, Italians were consuming twice as many grains as Americans, except for the last six years of the study when they dropped to less than double, but still remained substantially higher than the Americans.[10]

While the consumption of red meat in the U.S. was consistently greater than in Italy, the two countries differed in the way they used it. This difference in the amount of red meat consumed persisted despite the fact that the Italians more than doubled their use of meat during the thirty-year period, and beginning in the early 1970s, the Americans dropped theirs by 14 percent. Red meat was still the leading source of protein in the U.S., providing about 25 percent of the daily value, whereas in Italy the leading source of protein was grains. The protein contribution from poultry increased in both countries, and while fish was being consumed at about the same level in both countries at the start of the study period, by 1986 fish consumption had become 21 percent higher in Italy than in the U.S.

The Italian per-capita consumption of cheese, non-citrus fruits, tomatoes, other vegetables, and oils were all substantially higher than in the U.S. The Italians used more than twice the amount of oil, predominantly olive oil at first, but by 1986 the use of other vegetable oils accounted for more than half the total oil used in Italy. In the United States, the use of fats (butter, margarine, shortening, and lard) was initially more than four times that used in Italy, but as Italians increased their use of fats, the difference narrowed to twice the amount.

Not surprisingly, Italians ate two to three times as many tomatoes as Americans, and they ate 34 percent larger quantities of vegetables, including artichokes, cucumbers, eggplants, and cauliflower, than the Americans. The consumption of dark-green and deep-yellow vegetables was similar, and increased in both countries. Eating of sweet corn was standard in the U.S. but negligible in Italy. At the start of the study period, Italians were eating 60 percent more non-citrus fruits—apples, bananas, cantaloupes, cherries, grapes, peaches, pears, plums, strawberries, and watermelons—than Americans, and although that figure had dropped by 1986, they were still 28 percent higher. Figs and persimmons were regularly eaten in Italy, while pineapples were favored in the U.S. At the start of the study period, Americans ate 60 percent more citrus fruit than Italians, but as Italians increased their intake, the difference dwindled to 8 percent by 1986. Grains contributed more than half the carbohydrates for Italians, followed by sugars and sweeteners. Initially, the grains, sugars, and sweeteners contributed almost equally to the carbohydrate intake in the United States, but by 1986, the major source of this nutrient was grains, followed by sugars and sweeteners. Sweeteners were used twice as much in the U.S. as in Italy, and this difference persisted throughout the study period.

Based on their comparative analysis of the two diets, the researchers concluded that a combination of foods in the right balance offers the most health benefits. The primary implication of the U.S./Italy diet comparison was that a successful adoption of dietary recommendations requires consumer access to affordable, health-promoting foods. The researchers noted an increase in the availability of fruits and grains, and a shift to lower-fat dairy products and leaner meat products in the U.S. over the course of the study. They also noted that the overall U.S. food supply contained fewer dairy products, more sugar and sweeteners, and more fats and oils in 1986–1992 than in 1961–1965.

The researchers concluded that the idealized Mediterranean diet was the one that existed in Italy in the 1960s and not the one in practice three decades later. The Italian food supply in the 1960s had less milk, cheese, eggs, fats, meat, chicken, fish, sugars, sweeteners, and citrus fruits, and had more oils, grains, non-citrus fruits, white potatoes, tomatoes, and dark green, deep yellow, and other vegetables. In 1989–1992, the Italian food supply had more fats and oils, as well as more fruits, vegetables, and dairy products than in 1961–1965. Trends that deviated from the traditional Mediterranean diet in Italy were the decreased use of grains and increased use of red meats, sugars, and sweeteners.

A different study undertaken by a group of academic institutions and the National Research Council of Italy revealed that even older rural Italians are not following the traditional Mediterranean diet all that closely.[11] The purpose of the study was to describe the food-consumption patterns in an older rural population by estimating average daily intakes of carbohydrates, proteins, fats, minerals, and vitamins, and to assess the nutritional adequacy of these food patterns. Participants were drawn from two provinces, Pavia in Northern Italy and Cosenza in Southern Italy, to represent two areas where the dietary habits differed considerably. The Northern Italian diet is described as more continental, and the Southern Italian diet as more Mediterranean. The study's participants, 1465 women and 847 men, aged sixty-five years or older, were divided into groups as small eaters (eaters of a light diet), balanced-diet eaters, and those whose diets included larger than average amounts of cheese, alcohol, or coffee.

The balanced-diet group consisted of individuals with a low consumption of animal fats, oil, and alcoholic beverages, a moderate intake of cheese, meats and pasta, and a higher consumption of fruit, vegetables, and legumes. They also had the greatest fiber content in their diet. The researchers concluded this is the only group of people who came close to eating a Mediterranean diet. The small eaters came in second in their adherence to a Mediterranean diet, and consisted of those with a moderate intake of fish, low-fat meats, vegetables, pasta, and olive oil, and a below-average intake of dairy products. The others were found to deviate from the Mediterranean diet in varying degrees.

Given that the Mediterranean diet is characterized by a high intake of olive oil, fruits, and vegetables, the researchers concluded that the dietary habits of older Italians combined the typical elements of the Mediterranean diet with those of the *wealthy* diet (high in fats and sugars, low in complex carbohydrates) characteristic of Western countries. Notwithstanding the regional differences in food habits, the research revealed that such factors as education, physical activity, age, living status, and the degree of disability predicted the dietary behavior.

■ BRAZIL

Developing countries are undergoing diet transitions, leading them further from their traditional diets and closer to the diets prevalent in the richer countries with more meats and dairy products. One increasingly apparent consequence of such transitions is a rise in the incidence of diet-related diseases in those populations, adding to the burden of already existing health problems. Rice and beans, the traditional backbone of the Brazilian diet, provided several nutritional and health benefits. Leguminous diets that contain significant amounts of slowly absorbed carbohydrates have been shown to keep a person feeling full for longer periods of time and help prevent weight gain. Beans also serve as the main source of fiber in the Brazilian diet. But a steady decline in the consumption of legumes, accompanied by an increase in the consumption of such foods as meat and dairy products has been reported in Brazil. The ongoing nutritional transition in Brazil from their more traditional dietary pattern to a Western-type dietary pattern has been linked to an increase in the overall prevalence of overweight and obesity (body mass index of 30 or higher), reported to have gone from 2.5 percent in 1975 to 4.8 in 1989 among men, and from 6.9 percent to 11.7 among women. This rise in obesity rates occurred in spite of only a small increase in fat intake, from 26 percent to 28 percent during that period.[12]

In a 2002 study, researchers examined the dietary patterns of adult men and women and their associations with body weight in 2,000 households in Rio de Janeiro. They used body mass index (BMI) to differentiate between normal body weight, overweight, and obesity. The researchers tested the hypothesis that a traditional diet, based on rice and beans, would be protective against obesity among adults. A food-frequency questionnaire with eighty items and normal portions of the most regularly consumed foods was developed for the Brazilian population. The eighty items were collapsed into sixteen groups for analysis: rice, beans, cereals, eggs, deep-fried snacks, colas/sodas, coffee, juices, vegetables, milk products, margarine and butter, fruits, meat/pork/chicken, fish/shrimp, sweets, and alcohol. Using seven categories, the questionnaire asked participants to estimate the frequency of food consumption in the previous twelve months, ranging from three or more times per day, to less than once a month, and never, or almost never, and the portions of food intake in each category.[13]

At the time of the study, more than one-third of the adult population between the ages of twenty and sixty was overweight, and 12 percent were obese. The percentage of underweight and overweight were approximately the same in the three major ethnic groups studied, black, white, and mixed race. Forty-five percent of the participants reported a monthly per-capita income below U.S. $201 and 16 percent reported income above U.S. $600. Three major dietary patterns were identified: one that relied mainly on rice and beans—a traditional diet; a Western diet where fat (butter and margarine) and added sugar (sodas) were more often present, with infrequent consumption of rice and beans; and a mixed pattern where items from both the traditional and Western-type diets were consumed.

Among men, the Western diet included deep-fried snacks and milk products. More than 20 percent of the women and 10 percent of the men were on a weight-loss diet at the time of the survey. After adjusting for dieting, age, leisure time, physical activity, and occupation, only the traditional diet was found to have a lower risk of overweight and obesity, and a lower body mass index (BMI) overall. When participants were grouped by age into those between the ages of twenty and forty and those between forty-one and sixty, the association between the traditional diet and a lower risk of overweight or obesity was found only in the younger age group. The possibility that the middle-aged individuals had a more traditional diet that did not contain the higher-fat elements from the Western-type diet is given as a possible explanation for this outcome.

The protective role of the Brazilian traditional diet may be due to the low glycemic index of beans that keeps you feeling full for a longer period, and a reduced variety of the traditional diet. Rice and beans contribute to the bulk of the traditional Brazilian diet, which is also a low-fat diet. Fat intake has been considered a risk factor for weight gain in many studies across populations. Although there was a striking increase in obesity in Brazil, a high-fat intake was not reported, leading researchers to suspect that underreporting of fat intake as a possible reason why fat intake was not predictive of obesity in that country. After comparing responses given in the food-frequency questionnaire, more women than men were found to underestimate their fat intake, which led the researchers to conclude that a large group of participants were indeed underreporting their fat intake.

Based on the findings from Rio de Janeiro, the researchers concluded that the traditional combination of rice and beans as the major staple is protective against obesity.

■ CHINA

Although the Chinese are not exclusively vegetarians, their diet contains far more plant-based foods and substantially less meat and meat products than the typical Western diet. To put the proportions of plant- and animal-based foods in the two diets in perspective, the average intake of animal protein by the Chinese is one-tenth of the average intake in the United States. In 1983–1984, the Institute of Nutrition and Food Hygiene of the Chinese Academy of Preventive Medicine conducted a large nationwide survey of the dietary and lifestyle characteristics of 6,500 people in sixty-five, mostly rural, counties geographically scattered across China and their findings supported this preference for a variety of plant-based foods in the diet. A detailed three-day food history was collected from each individual in the study, and blood was drawn for measuring levels of cholesterol, iron, and hemoglobin. The men who participated in this study weighed 65 kg, were between eighteen and forty-five-years-old, and performed light physical activity. The information gathered was combined with mortality rates for several types of cardiovascular diseases, cancers, and communicable diseases, and was all published in 1991. Even if it's a bit dated, this is the most comprehensive diet and lifestyle study available from China, and researchers in the fields of epidemiology, nutrition, and public health regard it as a gold mine of data. Many performed secondary analyses on it, with specific attention paid to diet and chronic degenerative diseases in China. Colin Campbell at Cornell University's Division of Nutritional Sciences, and his collaborator Junshi Chen of the Institute of Nutrition and Food Hygiene of the Chinese Academy of Preventive Medicine reviewed a selection of publications containing analyses of the Chinese data and published a report of their findings in the *American Journal of Clinical Nutrition.*[14]

The sharp differences in the characteristics and diet composition of the people in rural China and those in the United States, in terms of body weight and height for the men and women; the intake of total protein, fiber, fat, and other nutrients; and the blood levels of cholesterol, iron, and hemoglobin, had already been well-documented in previously published reports. Relative to the rural Chinese, the intake of total protein and dietary fat were significantly higher among people in the United States. Due to the differences in population characteristics and the diet of the two countries, the researchers warned against sweeping conclusions about the diet/disease relationships found among residents of rural China and residents of highly industrialized societies like the U.S. The far lower consumption of dietary fat by the rural Chinese—14.5 percent vs. 38.8 percent by Americans—is reportedly achieved by a lower intake of foods of animal origin and a correspondingly higher intake of foods of plant origin, coupled with minimal addition of dietary fat. The total animal protein as a proportion of total protein intake among the Chinese is 10.8 percent, compared with 69 percent among the Americans.

Obesity is much less prevalent in China than the U.S. The average body mass index (BMI) for adult men in China is 20.5, while the corresponding figure in the United States at the time of the study is

25.8 (it is currently higher). Two factors are believed to be responsible for the lower obesity rates in China.

1. Greater physical activity—the use of bicycles for transportation is a prime example.

2. Eating fewer animal-based foods and more plant-based foods.

The authors of the report compared the greater leanness of Chinese adults to the well-studied Western vegetarians, especially vegans. The extent to which a low-fat diet and foods of animal origin independently contribute to body leanness remains unclear.

With respect to a connection between diet and chronic degenerative diseases, the China study revealed a clustering of two disease groups, one associated with poverty, the second with affluence, with such chronic degenerative diseases as coronary heart disease and several cancers in the latter group. The researchers were able to positively correlate these with high blood cholesterol, resulting from diets rich in saturated fats from animal sources and lacking in fiber-rich foods, such as legumes, other vegetables, and fruits. This dietary pattern correlated with that of the Western populations, although the latter was associated with higher blood cholesterol. Cholesterol levels measured in the rural Chinese at the time of the survey were substantially lower than levels found in the United States. This study showed that, in China, even a small intake of meat and fat are associated with a modest elevation of cholesterol levels, leading to coronary heart disease and other Western-type degenerative diseases, which suggests there is no threshold for cholesterol before it causes disease. The positive association between higher cholesterol levels and the prevalence of coronary heart disease seen in this study has been well documented worldwide for decades.

The China study also showed blood cholesterol levels to be directly associated with cancer mortality rates, and they were statistically significant for eight different cancers, including colon cancer. In general, the higher the cholesterol levels, the higher the risk of disease. The fat intake, although exceptionally low in comparison to Westerners, correlated weakly but positively with breast cancer. This is in spite of the fact that Chinese women, when compared with British women, were shown to start their periods later, experience menopause at an earlier age, have their first child at an earlier age, and have lower circulating concentrations of estrogen, all of which favor a lower risk for beast cancer. In the case of liver cancer, which is very prevalent in many parts of China, chronic infection with the hepatitis-B virus and cholesterol concentration are identified as the two main correlates. This is an uncommon finding because the usual suspect is *aflatoxin,* a carcinogen believed to cause human liver cancer, was not found to be the cause. This led the authors to suggest that the combination of chronic liver infection with the hepatitis-B virus, coupled with even a small elevation in cholesterol is sufficient to cause liver cancer. The average fiber intake in China is about three times higher than in the U.S. Although the association was not strong in this study, the death rates for colon and rectal cancer are consistently shown to be inversely correlated with the consumption of fiber and complex-carbohydrates. The findings of this landmark Chinese diet and disease survey led the authors to draw these conclusions.

1. Substantial decreases in intakes of dietary fat and animal protein and substantial increases in dietary fiber and other complex carbohydrates should result in continuing reductions in cholesterol levels and the associated chronic degenerative diseases.

2. Dietary measures to reduce the risk for chronic degenerative diseases would not necessarily result in increases in other adverse health effects, as long as the food choices are varied, the food is of good quality, and adequate in amount.

3. A diet rich in foods of plant origin can beneficially modify the risk for cancer and cardiovascular diseases.

■ INDIA

India's population exceeded one billion in 2001, and is expected to reach 1.33 billion by 2016. The Indian Government and the Food and Agriculture Organization (FAO) of the United Nations jointly reviewed the effects of the ongoing demographic changes in India in recent years—the rise and rates of urbanization, the trends in obesity and chronic-disease patterns between rural and urban communities, and the corresponding changes in diet and lifestyle.

A startling conclusion of that review is that the demographic changes in India, coupled with the changes in diet and lifestyle, is fueling an epidemic of obesity and chronic diseases, particularly in the urban areas. Dietary deficits and excesses, as well as the lifestyle changes that accompany industrialization and urbanization are believed to be responsible for the rising rates of obesity and the accompanying non-communicable diseases in India. This health and disease transition is resulting in chronic degenerative diseases that are now substituting for infectious and communicable diseases as the primary causes of morbidity and mortality. The review also points to the similarities between the Indian experience with non-communicable diseases and other developing countries, particularly those in rapid transition, such as Brazil and China.[15]

A major feature of the developmental transition in India is the rapid urbanization and the large shifts in population from rural to urban areas. The process of urbanization, although it differs greatly from state to state, is unrelenting and its consequences are staggering. Studies of migrant populations demonstrate that they adopt the diet, lifestyle patterns, and socio-cultural practices of the indigenous people, which result in their acquiring disease patterns similar to those of the native population. Similar variations in the risks for disease are seen within a country or region following internal rural-to-urban migration. Significant rural/urban differences in non-insulin-dependent diabetes mellitus and coronary heart disease rates exist in all regions of India, suggesting that internal migration, urbanization, and exposure to changing diet and lifestyles increase the risk of chronic disease.

As developing societies like India industrialize and urbanize, and as standards of living continue to rise, weight gain and obesity are beginning to pose a growing threat to the health of their citizens. Many experts say that an increase in fat intake, along with a decrease in levels of physical activity, is largely to blame. Lifestyle changes resulting in physical inactivity and sedentary behavior are important in contributing to obesity in children as well. This is exemplified by children spending more time in physically passive behaviors, such as watching television, playing video games, working on a computer, and talking on the telephone, similar to what children in the more advanced, Western countries are doing.

A report from the Nutrition Foundation of India reveals that the prevalence of obesity varies with the socio-economic status in urban India.[16]

The highest rates were found among the upper class (32.2 percent in men, 50 percent in women), followed by the middle class (16.2 percent in men, 30.3 percent in women), and the lower socio-economic groups (7.0 percent in men, 27.8 percent in women), and was least prevalent among the poor in urban slums (1.0 percent in men, 4.0 percent in women). The increase in the availability of food in developing countries is also accompanied by changes in the diet. Data from the Food and Agriculture Organization (FAO) show that the changes in Asian countries, including India, has been relatively small, but there have been large changes in the consumption of animal products, sugars, and fats.[17] Data from India show that the diet of higher-income groups had 32 percent of it coming from fat, while only 17 percent came from fat in the lower income groups. A study of obesity among the adults in Delhi confirms that the upper-income groups in urban India currently consume higher levels of fat compared with the urban poor or rural populations.[18]

A study in Mumbai showed that the prevalence of obesity among young adult males varied from 10.7 percent to 53.1 percent. A large study from urban Delhi, however, showed the overall prevalence of obesity to be 27.8 percent, with a higher prevalence (33.4 percent) among women.[19] The Delhi study also indicated that obesity was associated with raised levels of circulating cholesterol and fats in the blood, and lower levels of physical activity. A more recent report on adults over age forty from the State of Kashmir showed the overall prevalence of obesity to be 15.0 percent, with a higher prevalence among women (23.7 percent vs. 7.0 percent among men). The true prevalence of obesity in India is difficult to estimate, as it can be under- or overestimated in the published reports. Nevertheless, it is indisputable that the problem of obesity, at least in the urban population, is on the rise in India. Obesity, both in children and adults, and its contribution to non-communicable chronic diseases, is likely to become a serious health problem in India, with economic development and urbanization altering dietary habits and lifestyle patterns.

There have been many nationally representative surveys on patterns of diet, nutrition, and food consumption in India since the 1970s. They all showed a gradual increase in caloric intake, typified by an increase in consumption of cereal grains, while the intake of most other foods, including milk, oil, and sugar, remained largely unchanged. However, many of these surveys revealed disparities between rural and urban populations and between different socio-economic groups. Comparison of food-consumption patterns shows a gradual reduction in cereal-grain consumption between 1975 and 1995. This is largely the result of a progressive increase in the intake of protein, and probably fats—the latter due to a large increase in the consumption of milk and milk products, and an increase in the intake of meat, fats, and oils. The consumption of legumes has fallen dramatically as the production of several of the legumes has not kept pace with the rise in population, and the demand for exports. This is a cause for much concern since legumes are a very important source of proteins in the typical Indian diet.

Food balance data from the FAO show India at the bottom of the group of countries with a fat-calorie ratio just over 15 percent, a total fat intake at 37.8 grams per day, and a 27.5 percent animal fat to total fat ratio.[20] Trends show that the per-capita supply of animal products has increased by more than 60 percent between 1965 and 1999. Improvement in socio-economic status is also often associated with reduced consumption of coarse cereal grains as a preference for the highly polished varieties with much lower dietary fiber increases. Most plant-based foods are generally good sources of vitamins, minerals, and fiber, as well as phytochemical compounds. The area of cultivation and food production has increased dramatically over the years in India, and as a result the country has gained a prominent share in the global production of fruits and vegetables. The native population, however, does not reflect this in an increased consumption of fruits and vegetables, possibly due to the emphasis on cash crops for export and sale.

Declining physical activity as a result of the increasing mechanization of work, increased urbanization, greater use of cars and motorcycles, more leisure time, often spent passively watching television, have all contributed to an inevitable weight gain among men, women, and to a lesser extent in children, in India. This, in turn, is spiking the rates of such conditions as heart disease, adult-onset diabetes, and cancer. Chronic disease first affects the affluent classes in a population and then percolates through to other social classes over time; this is something seen in industrialized societies decades ago that is now being manifested in rapidly developing countries like India.

■ SOUTH AFRICA

The South African population is predominantly black, comprising 77.4 percent of the total populace, and is also the most impoverished of all groups living in that country. While more than half the blacks live in non-urban areas, the proportion of people calling urban- and peri-urban (fringes of cities) areas home has steadily increased to a little more than 40 percent. South Africa is bearing a quadruple burden of disease—poverty-related infectious disease, the burgeoning HIV/AIDS epidemic, lifestyle-related non-communicable diseases, and violence-related trauma. As in other developing countries, diet and physical inactivity that contribute to the development of chronic diseases in South Africa have garnered much attention in recent years. Rural/urban comparisons of African populations have led many academics to believe that the urban exposure is causing the traditional African diet to be replaced by a Western-type diet, typically high in fat and low in carbohydrates and dietary fiber, and associated with an increased prevalence of degenerative diseases. This, in fact, was borne out by several nationally representative surveys done in South Africa in the past two decades.

A 1990 study of men and women fifteen to sixty-four years old, living in Cape Town, South Africa, correlated diet with years of urban exposure, determined from migration history.[21] The findings reveal that fat intake increased significantly, and there was a corresponding decrease in carbohydrate intake with urban dwelling in South Africa. Also notable was a significant increase in animal protein in the diet of the newly urbanized, with a corresponding decrease in plant protein. Data on diet and length of urban residence obtained from black adults in the city of Johannesburg also showed even more pronounced shifts in fat and carbohydrate intake. These changes in diet are more dramatic than those observed in Western countries undergoing industrialization over longer periods of time. The proportion of fat and carbohydrates obtained by black South Africans did meet the requirements of the South African Diet Consensus Panel, which are also consistent with the American Heart Association's recommendations. It does, however, represent a transitional phase between the traditional diet (60 percent from carbohydrates, 25 percent from fat) and a Western eating pattern (50 percent from carbohydrates, 35 percent from fats). Large percentages of people in the South African survey fell below two-thirds of the Recommended Dietary Allowance (RDA) for several vitamins and minerals, reflecting a nutritionally depleted diet. As well, the participants were consuming less than half the recommended dairy per day. The recommended minimum of four portions of fruits and vegetables was consumed by only 50 percent of the population, with a quarter of the respondents not reporting any.

The Cape Town study revealed that the newer arrivals to the city are generally associated with low educational status, inadequate housing, and diets low in fat but also lacking in vitamins and minerals. Their more urbanized counterparts, with a higher educational status and living in formal housing, consumed diets somewhat richer in micronutrients, but also significantly higher in fats and lower in carbohydrates. These differences in diets between those who have taken up residence in urban areas for some time and those who have just set foot in an urban area leads to questioning if improvements in socio-economic status are bringing about a shift to a nutritional pattern that predisposes people to chronic diseases. Many factors affect food choices and methods of food preparation. Poverty, a lack of knowledge, and social instability in the black population keep healthy eating from being a priority in the minds of township dwellers. The authors of these studies point out that the long commuting distances of employed city dwellers frequently result in choosing easy-to-prepare foods, and eating snacks away from home, which are generally high in refined sugars, and high in fat content. Conversely, the more traditionally orientated individuals are frequently the under-employed newer arrivals who may have the time to prepare relatively low-cost maize- and legume-based dishes, which require longer cooking times. In addition to the changes in nutritional patterns over time and the degree of urbanization that black South Africans are undergoing, women with no education were found to have a lower mean body mass index (BMI) than those with schooling. The difference is explained by the fact that these women were engaged in occupations that involved more manual labor than their better-educated counterparts.[22] Although high rates of obesity were reported among Africans, fewer than 5 percent of the men and 15 percent of the women perceived themselves as obese. Increasing urbanization and a rise in socio-economic status in developing populations appear to increase their partiality to a Western-style diet, along with greater inactivity, obesity, and the associated consequences of such diseases as hypertension, diabetes, and strokes. The rise of these chronic diseases of lifestyle origin poses a considerable challenge for South Africa, as it needs to balance its resources among the quadruple burdens mentioned earlier.

■ UNITED STATES

The typical American diet tends to be high in meat and saturated fat, and low in fruits, vegetables, and whole grains. Meat and dairy foods contribute all the dietary cholesterol and the great majority of saturated fat. The average American derives 67 percent of dietary protein from animal sources, compared with a worldwide average of 34 percent. The average U.S. consumption of meat is 222 pounds per person per year. Despite the negative publicity it has garnered in recent decades, red meat continues to be a top-choice main course in the American diet.[23]

The animal-feeding operations system provides artificially cheap meat for the consumer, and consumer demand, in turn, fuels this system of meat production. In the United States before 1850, virtually all cattle were free-range or pasture-fed, and were typically slaughtered at four to five years of age. By about 1885, the science of rapidly fattening cattle in feedlots had advanced to the point that it was possible to produce a 545-kilo steer ready for slaughter in twenty-four months.[24]

The amount of meat and saturated fat consumed in the U.S. clearly exceeds nutritional needs. The six major sources of saturated fats in the American diet are fatty meats, baked goods, cheese, milk, margarine, and butter. Substantial evidence now indicates that in order to prevent the risk of chronic disease, the absolute amount of dietary fat is less important than the type of fat. Monounsaturated fats and some polyunsaturated fats are beneficial to health, where as most saturated fats and trans fats are detrimental to health when consumed in excessive quantities.

The rising prevalence of overweight and obesity in the U.S. among all age groups and both genders has caused attention to be focused on the eating behavior of Americans. A number of studies have examined nutrient intake, particularly fat. A group of researchers at the University of North Carolina, Chapel Hill, examined the intake related to eating locations and the consumption of certain key food items between 1977 and 1996. They used the data from four large, nationally representative surveys of the U.S. population older than age two. For each food consumed in all four surveys, the participant (or the caregiver) was asked whether this was a meal or a snack, and where the food was eaten. The researchers found a significant increase in the percentage of food eaten away from home, specifically from restaurants and fast-food eateries. In the process, Americans increased their consumption of sugars significantly. There was also a much larger relative increase in snacks eaten, rather than meals, during the same period. Snacks represented a larger portion of the diets of those between ages two and eighteen than the diets of other age groups. The largest increases were in consumption of salty snacks, soft drinks, and pizza. Consumption of candy, fruit drinks,

French fries, cheeseburgers, and Mexican food also increased for all age groups but accounted only for a small percentage of the total diet, and the changes over time were small.[25]

A 2009 Diet and Health study, conducted by the National Institutes of Health (NIH) and the American Association of Retired Persons (AARP), examined how meat consumption affects mortality.[26] This large study of more than half a million men (59 percent) and women (41 percent), between the ages of fifty and seventy-one years, evaluated the association between the overall death rate and the consumption of three categories of meat—red meat, including all cuts of beef and pork; white meat, consisting of poultry and fish; and processed meats like bacon, cold cuts, ham, hot dogs, luncheon meats, and sausages. Based on their findings, the researchers concluded that the men who ate the most red meat had a 31-percent higher death rate than those men who ate the least. A consumption of processed meat was associated with a 16-percent higher death rate. The latter is particularly significant because the participants consumed only an average of 1.5 ounces of processed meat a day. A high intake of white meat (poultry and fish) was associated with a reduced rate of death among both men and women. The deaths from cardiovascular disease and cancer followed the same pattern as total deaths, and women were affected similarly to men.

The results of the study held up even after the researchers took into account other health habits and risk factors among the participants. The findings of the NIH-AARP study, one of the largest of its kind, are also supported by earlier studies that had established a strong link between consumption of red meat and cancer, colon cancer in particular. While scientists are not certain why eating red meat increases the risk of colon cancer, two culprits are suspected—heterocyclic amines, the chemicals produced when meat is cooked at high temperatures, and the N-nitroso compounds (NOCs) used as preservatives in processed meats and converted by the body into nitrosamines, which are known carcinogens.

The fiber content of the typical U.S. diet (15.1 grams per day) is considerably lower than recommended values (25–30 grams per day). Refined sugars, vegetable oils, dairy products, and alcohol do not contain any fiber, and they are prevalent in the typical American diet. Refined grains make up the bulk of the grains (85 percent) consumed in the United States, and these contain only a small fraction of the fiber present in unrefined whole grains, thus diluting the total dietary fiber intake. A one-half-cup serving of most legumes provides a sub-stantial percentage (25–30 percent) of the recommended value of fiber in the diet. The USDA recommended (but not followed) serv-ings of fresh fruits and vegetables not only provide the much-needed fiber, but also contain valuable micronutrients like the vitamins and minerals. Furthermore, widely available processed foods—bagels, baked goods (cakes and cookies, etc.), breakfast cereals, candy, chips, condiments, crackers, ice cream, muffins, pizza, rolls, salad dressings, and soft drinks—contain little or no fiber, but tend to be a regular part of the typical American diet.

Food portions in the U.S. have also been steadily increasing, both at home and when eating out. Nationally representative data from four large surveys by the Nationwide Food Consumption Survey (1977–1978) and the Continuing Survey of Food Intake by Individu-als (1989–1991, 1994–1996, and 1998) have all pointed to this trend. Between 1977 and 1996, portion sizes and energy intake for all key foods (except pizza) increased at all locations for the total U.S. pop-ulation, aged two years and older. The sizes of portions were found to vary depending on where people ate, with the largest increase in portions consumed at fast-food restaurants and the smallest at other restaurants.

Portion sizes for certain foods increased more than others. Between 1977 and 1996, the portion size of salty snacks increased from 1.0 to 1.6 ounces (from 132 to 225 kcal), the average size of soft drinks con-sumed increased from 13.1 to 19.9 fluid ounces (from 144 to 193 kcal), and the average cheeseburger went from 5.8 to 7.3 ounces (from 397 to 533 kcal). High-fat beef and pork consumption decreased substan-tially across all age groups, and high-fat luncheon meat and hot-dog intake decreased slightly. Overall, in this twenty-year period, Ameri-cans doubled their intake of cheeseburgers, French fries, hamburg-ers, Mexican food, pizza, and sugared drinks with the meals. The differences between groups were very small, the only substantial one being that the intake of alcohol as a snack was much higher in men than in women.[27]

Ultimately, what makes Americans eat what they do? To what extent do taste, nutrition, cost, convenience, and calories influence the choice of foods Americans consume? This is precisely the subject of two surveys conducted by a group of researchers on a national sample of nearly 3,000 people. The focus of the surveys was consumption of breakfast cereals, cheese, fast foods, and fruits and vegetables. The results were published in the *Journal of the American Dietetic Association*, and they showed clear demographic variations in how important taste, nutrition, cost, convenience, and weight-control concerns are to individuals. Regardless of age, income level, and ethnicity, taste was universally rated as the most important, making *tasting good* a minimal requirement for choosing a food. Cost and convenience were more important to younger people, while older people rated nutrition and weight control higher. In the surveys, women rated taste, nutrition, cost, and weight control higher than men did. Not surprisingly, people who said fast food is more convenient than fruits, vegetables, and breakfast cereals were more likely to eat fast food more often. Greater concerns about nutrition and weight control were associated with those who ate more fruits and vegetables and less fast food.[28]

A better understanding of the changing diets of Americans is gained by looking both at key foods and the location where they are eaten. The most significant trend is clearly the continued shift from home to away from home. Today, the average American consumes 65 percent of his or her food at home, representing a 12-percent decline from twenty years before. The results of the surveys contradict the general perception that the major shifts in eating behavior are among the young. Although there are differences in the amounts of foods consumed and the location of foods consumed by age, these differences have remained constant over the past twenty years. This dispels the idea that certain age groups are increasing their intake disproportionately, including, for example, the perception that the explosion of soft drinks or French fries was only among teenagers or other selected groups. Across the board, the incidence of foods eaten outside the home is increasing and is possibly contributing to the increase in obesity. This raises the possibility that our whole environment is changing, not just the actions of certain individuals.

Americans have increased their overall consumption over the past twenty years, the largest increase being in sugared beverages. The most important relative decreases have been in milk and meat products eaten alone. It is apparent that people of all ages are making unhealthy choices both inside and, especially, outside the home. Although there have been some positive changes, including decreased consumption of red meats, there seem to be many other components of the American diet that need to be modified. One important way of changing people's eating behavior is to encourage them to eat at home more and to make healthier choices when eating out. Consumers need to be encouraged to eat more fruits and vegetables and fewer high-fat refined-grain dishes. It is hoped that if people change their diets to include more healthy food inside and outside the home, the rise in obesity will be curbed, along with the accompanying incidences of chronic disease.

In the United States, cancer, diabetes, heart disease, and other chronic diseases attributable to diet and lifestyle represent the most serious threat to public health by far. Two-thirds of the adult population over age twenty in the United States is either overweight (more than 20 percent above the normal weight) or obese (BMI of 30 or greater). Heart disease continues to be the number-one cause of death among both men and women, despite a modest decline in recent years. Cancer is the second leading cause of death, contributing to a quarter of all deaths in the United States. Adult-onset diabetes, so called because it has typically affected adults over the age of forty, is now being seen in children. In 2001, metabolic syndrome, a new disease classification representing a cluster of cardiovascular risk factors triggered primarily by overweight and obesity, was formally added to the International Classification of Diseases (ICD-9) as a disease category. The growing awareness of the high costs imposed on society by the rising incidence of diet-related diseases provides a strong case for policies to promote a healthy diet that is well diversified between foods of animal and plant origin and contains recommended amounts of macro and micro nutrients and fiber.

THE EXPERIENCES OF THESE DIVERSE POPULATIONS CAN SERVE AS LESSONS

Diet-related chronic diseases represent the single largest cause of morbidity and mortality in the U.S. and other industrialized countries. The less industrialized countries that are experiencing rapid urbanization and changes in socioeconomic conditions are increasingly adopting elements of the Western-type diet rich in such foods as meats, fats, and sugars. As a result, they too are now experiencing rising rates of overweight and obesity accompanied by a rise in chronic diseases like heart disease, adult-onset diabetes and certain cancers. The worldwide demand for animal foods will continue to increase as the population grows, and rising incomes allow urban elites everywhere to adopt the high-meat, high-fat diet now typical in the U.S.

Perhaps the lesson here is that the time has come for the U.S. and other more industrialized countries to serve as role models, scaling back on meats, fats, and sugars, and replacing some of their animal-based foods with plant-based ones. And certainly legumes, lean-protein, high-fiber, and micronutrient-rich foods deserve a prominent place in the plant-based food category. Including a variety of animal- and plant-based foods in your diet can not only ensure that you're getting all the necessary nutrients, but can also lessen the likelihood of overloading on harmful foods. And this, in turn, might send a strong signal to the less industrialized world to stop mimicking the Western diet.

🐟 5 🐟

Most Commonly Eaten Legumes in the U.S. and Around the World

THE COMMON BEAN

Many of the dry beans—red/kidney beans, pinto beans, black beans, white/navy beans, cannellini beans, among them—are referred to as the common bean because they all belong to one legume family whose botanical name is *Phaseolus vulgaris*. They are all believed to have originated in Peru. The largest commercial producers of dried common beans today are Brazil, China, India, Indonesia, and the United States. Because these beans are also among the most popularly known and consumed legumes, they merit individual descriptions here.

■ RED/KIDNEY BEAN

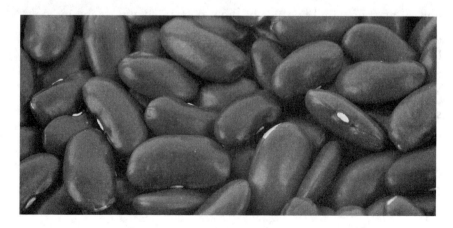

Kidney beans, so called because their shape resembles that of a kidney, most probably originated in Peru, and were spread throughout South and Central America by migrating Peruvian Indian traders. Spanish explorers returning from their voyages to the New World introduced them into Europe in the fifteenth century, and Spanish and Portuguese traders subsequently brought these beans to Africa and Asia. Today, kidney beans are grown and consumed worldwide, Brazil and India being the largest producers.

The kidney bean is also known as the red bean (not to be confused with other red beans) and the chili bean because it is generally the bean of choice in preparing *chili con carne*—chili pepper with meat in Spanish—a popular, spicy stew-like dish. In local variations, it can be found worldwide, as well as in some American-style fast-food restaurants.

Both dried and canned kidney beans are available throughout the year. Dried beans are generally available pre-packaged in small quantities as well as in bulk bins. Prior to purchase, it is important to ensure that there is no evidence of moisture or insect damage and that the beans are whole and not cracked. Most grocery stores, the larger chain stores as well as the smaller specialty stores, carry canned kidney beans.

There is little difference between the nutritional value of canned kidney beans and those you cook yourself, with the exception of sodium content, which tends to be significantly higher in canned beans. If you are faced with a choice between using canned beans or not eating them at all because of the inconvenience involved in cooking the raw beans, choose the canned beans by all means, rather than forgo eating this richly nutritious and delicious food, but be sure to rinse them thoroughly before use to remove much of the added salt. Always read the label on the container to know the exact amount of sodium per serving and look for one that contains the least amount of added salt.

It's best to store raw kidney beans in an airtight container in a cool, dry, and dark place where they will keep for up to twelve months. Cooked kidney beans will keep in the refrigerator for about three days if placed in a covered container.

Nutritional Profile

One cup of cooked kidney beans contains 15 grams of protein, nearly a third of the recommended daily value (DV), 11 grams of fiber (45 percent of the DV), 5.2 milligrams of iron (29.5 percent of the DV) and 230 micrograms of the B vitamin folic acid (57 percent of the DV). Kidney beans also contain significant proportions of other vitamins and minerals, including copper, magnesium, phosphorus, potassium, thiamin (vitamin B_1), and vitamin K.

■ PINTO OR MOTTLED BEANS

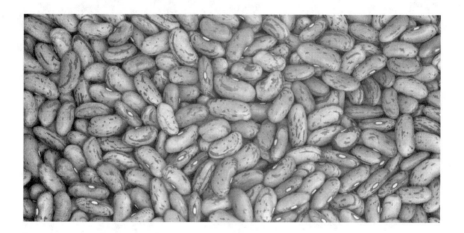

The pinto bean (in Spanish, *frijol pinto* means *painted bean*) is named for its mottled skin, as shown above. In the cooked form, the colored splotches that give the bean a mottled appearance disappear, leaving a smooth, pink color and a creamy texture. Pinto beans were spread throughout South and Central America, and later Europe, Asia, and Africa in the same way as kidney beans. Pinto beans are the most widely produced and consumed bean in the United States, and Dove Creek, Colorado, is regarded as the Pinto Bean Capital of the world. These beans were once a staple in the Southeastern United States, especially during the winter months. Some churches in rural areas of this region still sponsor pinto-bean suppers for social gatherings and fundraisers. The young pods of pinto beans may also be harvested and cooked.

Nutritional Profile

The nutritional power of the pinto bean, not unlike its peer the kidney bean, lies in its high protein content. One cup yields 16 grams of protein (31 percent of the DV), 5.5 grams of fiber (62 percent of the DV), low amounts of fat, significant percentages of several vitamins, plus minerals, calcium and iron in particular. It is worth noting that more than one half the calories in a cup of cooked pinto beans come from their protein content.

■ BLACK BEANS

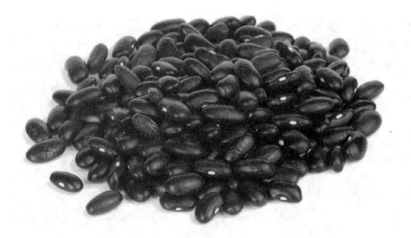

Black beans could not be more succinctly and descriptively named. They are generally referred to as turtle beans, probably due to their shiny, dark, shell-like appearance. With a rich flavor that has been compared to mushrooms, black beans have a velvety texture and hold their shape well during cooking. As one of the variety of common beans (*Phaseolus vulgaris*), black beans share many characteristics with their fellow bean-family members, including kidney beans, white/navy beans, yellow beans, pinto beans, pink beans, and Anasazi beans. Brazil grows more black beans than any country in the world. Designated as their own unique food group, beans have been given an exclusive place on the Brazilian Food Pyramid, and the *2006 Food Guide for the Brazilian Population* recommends that beans be consumed at least once every day. That recommendation is actually quite close to the *Dietary Guidelines for Americans,* which recommends 3 cups of cooked legumes per week, or a one-half cup serving six days per week, as the minimum desired amount. Recent research linking bean intake to a lowered risk of adult-onset diabetes, many types of cardiovascular disease, and several types of cancer was one of the key factors used by the Brazilian and U.S. governments to establish their bean-intake recommendations.

Nutritional Profile

Black beans are a star legume in terms of providing a significant proportion of daily values (DV) of protein and fiber. One cup of cooked black beans provides nearly a third of a day's requirement of protein, and nearly 60 percent of the recommended daily allowance (RDA) of dietary fiber. A quarter of the fiber in a cup (more than 4 grams) is soluble fiber, the type that researchers have found especially helpful in lowering blood cholesterol levels. A decreased risk of coronary heart disease (CHD), and myocardial infarction (MI, or heart attack) have both been associated with an increased intake of soluble fiber from food, in particular soluble fiber from legumes. Although brightly colored fruits and vegetables are generally regarded as the best sources of phytonutrients (plant nutrients), research on legumes has shown black beans to be a star contender in this arena.

Black beans are an outstanding source of three flavonoids that are primarily responsible for the rich black color seen on the bean's surface. They contain well-documented antioxidant and anti-inflammatory properties that serve as especially important protection for the cardiovascular system. Their role in preventing excessive chronic oxidative stress and chronic inflammation has been established as a key factor in decreasing the risk for most cardiovascular diseases and certain cancers, especially colon cancer.

Another important nutrient in black beans that provides cardiovascular benefits is folic acid, arguably one of the most important B vitamins for decreasing the risk of cardiovascular disease. One cup of black beans provides nearly two-thirds the daily value (DV) of this B vitamin. Black beans are also a rich source of magnesium, more frequently associated with cardiovascular protection than any other single mineral. One cup of cooked black beans provides about 120 milligrams or one-third of the DV for this mineral.

Finally, black beans provide about 180 milligrams of omega-3 fatty acids per cup in the form of alpha-linolenic acid (ALA). Being rich in protein and fiber content, black beans help move food from the stomach to the small intestine (a process known as gastric emptying) at a slower, more desirable pace than foods containing less of these nutrients and more sugars. This helps maintain blood sugar at a steady level instead of causing peaks and valleys in the bloodstream. The slower gastric emptying also keeps hunger in check between meals.

People often think of black beans, and beans in general, as intestinal-gas-producing food. However, research has shown that black beans contain a larger indigestible food fraction than some other beans, and this allows bacteria in the colon to produce butyric acid, which aids in better digestion of food in the colon, including sugars, thus minimizing gas production in the large intestine.

■ BLACK TURTLE BEANS

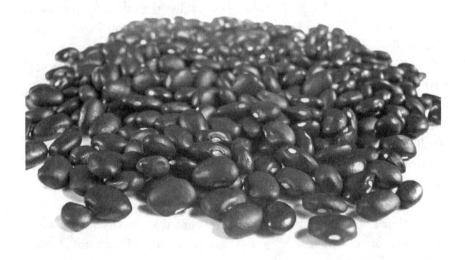

The black turtle bean is a smaller variety of the black bean with a shinier skin, and is especially popular in Latin American cuisine. It has a dense, meaty texture and flavor reminiscent of mushrooms, and is an extremely good source of nutritional antioxidants. It is a very frequently consumed bean in various regions of Brazil, and is also popular in Cuba, Costa Rica, Nicaragua, and Venezuela. The nutritional profile of black turtle beans is very similar to that of black beans.

■ WHITE/NAVY BEANS

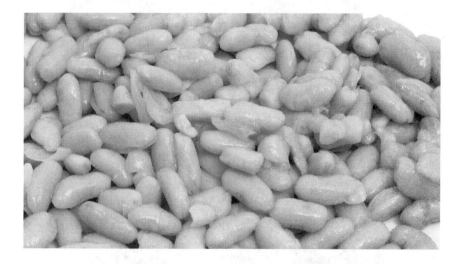

Navy beans are small, pea-sized beans that are creamy white in color. The bean got its current popular name *navy bean* because it was a staple food of the United States Navy in the early twentieth century. Cannellini, great Northern, and navy beans are three popular types of white beans. Navy beans are mild-flavored, dense, and creamy in texture, and are particularly popular in Britain and the U.S. Like other common beans, navy beans originated in Peru and took the same routes through South and Central America, Europe, Asia, and Africa. Today, the largest commercial producers of navy beans, along with other dried common beans, are Brazil, China, India, Indonesia, and the United States.

Nutritional Profile

The nutritional benefits of the navy bean come from its all-star status in fiber content (76 percent of the DV), the B vitamin folate (63 percent of DV), 30 percent DV of protein, and significant proportions of other vitamins and minerals, all in one cup of cooked beans.

■ CANNELLINI BEANS

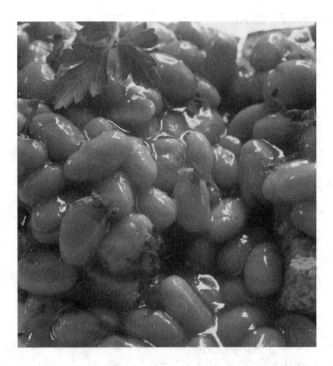

The Cannellini bean is a larger navy bean, and is kidney shaped, which is why it is also called a white kidney bean, or *haricot blanc* in French. These beans have a tender creamy flesh with a slightly nutty taste and a mild earthiness, and are considered one of the best white beans for salads and ragouts. Cannellini beans have a moderately thin skin that allows them to absorb flavors well, even as they hold their shape in cooking, both of which make them very versatile.

Nutritionally, cannellini beans are very similar to navy beans and are quite popular in the cuisine of Central and Southern Italy.

■ FAVA BEANS/ BROAD BEANS

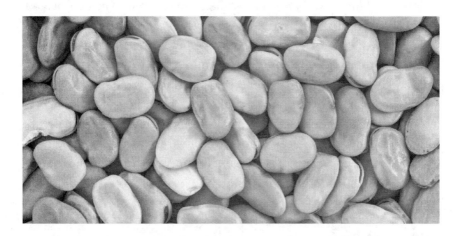

The term fava bean came from the Italian word *fava,* meaning broad, and is still known as a broad bean in several countries, including the United Kingdom, for its large-seeded pod. It is the fruit of an annual herbaceous plant believed by botanists to have originated in North Africa and the Mediterranean region. The plant is tall, with large leaves that do not have tendrils for climbing over other vegetation, causing the plant to grow erect. This tall, erect plant may very well be the bean plant referred to in the children's story *Jack and the Bean Stalk.* It is believed that, along with lentils, peas, and chickpeas, fava beans became part of the Eastern Mediterranean diet in or around 6000 BC.

These beans are said to have been cultivated in biblical times by the Hebrews and later by the Egyptians, the Greeks, and the Romans. Sicily is said to have once experienced a failure of all crops except fava beans, so Italians credit fava beans with keeping Sicilians from starvation during a time of famine. In return, thanks were given to Saint Joseph, and subsequently these beans were offered at the altar on St. Joseph Day. Since then, fava beans have been considered good luck in that part of Italy.

The Greeks used fava beans as ballots in voting and believed that souls could be reincarnated in this food. During Saturnalia celebrations in ancient Rome, the fava bean was used to designate the king of the banquet, a custom that may be at the origin of the use of a single bean in the traditional cake of the Twelfth Night celebrations. Fava-bean plants have been among the most ancient plants cultivated in Old World agriculture and are among the easiest to grow. The pod is broad and leathery, green in color when young, turning blackish-brown when matured. The beans have a buttery texture, slight bitterness, and a nutty flavor that some find lingering as an aftertaste.

Fava beans have two layers of shells. The external shell is removed before the beans are dried and packaged. Removing the shell surrounding the dried fava bean eliminates the gritty texture between the shell and the body of the fava bean. Removing the dried fava bean shell from the body requires loosening the bond that releases the skins from the beans.

Nutritional Profile

Fava beans are loaded with nutritional benefits. They are high in protein, fiber, folic acid, and iron, and are extremely low in fat. One cup of cooked beans provides 13 grams of protein, 33 grams of carbohydrates, 9 grams of fiber, 1 gram of fat, and only 187 calories. Additionally, fava beans are particularly rich in folic acid (a B vitamin), yielding 44 percent of the DV in one cup of cooked beans. Copper, manganese, and phosphorus are also key nutrients in fava beans. Fresh fava beans are low in sodium, but canned ones contain significantly more sodium (18 milligrams vs. 500 milligrams per cup).

■ LIMA BEANS

Lima beans are large, kidney-shaped, flat beans with a creamy texture and a sweetish flavor. As the name might suggest, they did originate in Lima, Peru, around 6000 BC, and belong to the *Phaseolus* bean family. Young lima beans are pale green (sold in stores as baby lima beans), and as they mature they develop a pale yellow color, which is the reason they are called butter beans in England and later in the Southern United States. The Italian name for these beans, *fagioli di spagna,* speaks to their Spanish connection, as Spanish colonists brought them to Italy. The beans also go by the name Madagascar beans because they are extensively cultivated on this island off the east coast of Africa. Lima beans can also be purple, red, brown, or black in color. Some varieties of lima beans are mottled and are referred to as speckled butter beans. The two primary varieties of lima beans are the fordhook and the smaller, milder-tasting, baby lima. Dried lima beans come packaged in storable bags, or canned and pre-cooked, while fresh ones are sold shelled, frozen, or raw in their pods.

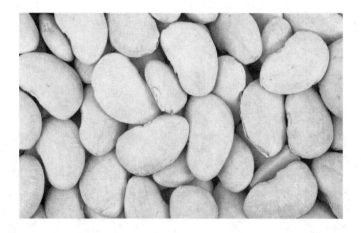

Heirloom and exotic varieties of lima beans are also sold in the market. Baby white lima beans, believed to be of Guatemalan or Mexican origin, are small, flat, cream-colored beans that are less mealy, with a milder, sweeter flavor than their larger peers. They are often mixed with sweet corn to make succotash, or added to vegetable soups. The Hopi orange lima bean, so called because it resembles an ancient orange bean found in Peru by the Hopi Indians who preserved this heirloom lima as a dry bean they ground for flour. Worcester Indian red pole limas, or simply red lima beans, were ground for flour or eaten together with red corn by Native Americans. In the Southern United States, slaves used to cook the beans with goober peas and red sweet potatoes to make *fufu* (African mashed dumplings). Christmas lima beans, so called because of their chestnut flavor, nutty texture, and dark red color with brown streaks that are retained even after cooking, were once very popular, and are still available from specialty companies that sell dry beans.

Nutritional Profile

The main nutritional benefits of lima beans lie in their fiber content (one cup of cooked lima beans provide nearly two-thirds of the daily requirement), manganese (48.5 percent DV) with its antioxidant properties, and iron (24.9 percent DV), essential for forming hemoglobin in the body.

■ SOYBEANS

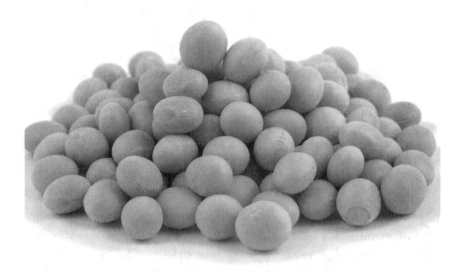

Soybeans belong to the plant family *Fabaceae,* which is native to East Asia, and are believed to have been used for thousands of years in China, where they probably originated. These beans are also very popular in Japan. Soybeans have been introduced to the Western world since the beginning of the twentieth century.

Soybeans grow in a variety of soils and a wide range of climates and have come to be known as the kingpins of legumes, both because of their extremely high nutritional value and their worldwide economic importance as a crop. There are more than a 1,000 varieties of this versatile legume, ranging in size and in color from yellow, green, and red, to black, white, and even mottled. Soy consumption is vastly different in the East and the West. When Westerners think of soybeans, they most likely picture soy sauce, the ubiquitous dark, salty liquid used to flavor Asian foods, but this is only one of many ways that soybeans are consumed worldwide. Surveys of soy consumption from China and Japan reveal an average consumption of 100–200 grams per day in those countries. The United States continues to be among the top producers of soybeans, although not their top consumer—the average soy consumption in the U.S. is less than one-tenth the amount in China and Japan. Because soybeans are used in processing many food products, especially in the United States, their consumption is indirect and difficult to quantify. In addition to their use for food, soybeans have diverse applications, such as ink for newspapers, and candles that burn cleaner than petroleum-based candles.

Nutritional Profile

Nutritionally, there is no other plant food that can measure up to soybeans, for they are the only plant food that is a complete protein, containing all eight essential amino acids. For this reason, soybeans have been dubbed the meat of the soil and the *miracle beans.* Other nutritional strengths of soybeans lie in their exceptionally low-carbohydrate and low-saturated-fat contents. One cup of soybeans contains as much protein as or more than 3 ounces of cooked meat, and contains none of the harmful saturated fats.

Despite soybean's being a nutritional giant, and inexpensive, the average American household does not consume this legume on a regular basis in amounts that would yield significant benefits. Following evidence from research pointing to the LDL-lowering benefit from soybean consumption, the Food and Drug Administration approved this health claim for soy, indicating that a daily consumption of 25 grams of soy protein may lower LDL cholesterol (the bad cholesterol). Since sprinkling a little soy sauce on your sushi rolls at the table is not sufficient to fully derive its benefits, it makes good nutritional sense to substitute animal protein with this plant protein a few times a week.

■ MUNG BEANS

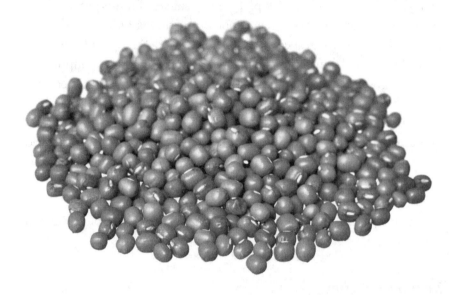

Mung beans, small, olive-green beans, are believed to have originated in India, where they continue to be among the most consumed legumes. Also called green grams, or golden grams, they are cultivated in several countries of Asia, Africa, and South America. In the U.S., mung beans are grown in areas that have sandy loam soils and dry conditions, such as Oklahoma and Missouri. But domestic production is not sufficient to keep pace with consumption, so nearly three-fourths of the mung beans consumed in the U.S. are imported. Mung-bean seeds range in color from green to brown, and are about half the diameter of soybean seeds. The beans have a slightly sweet flavor and soft texture. When their skin is removed and the beans are split, they are a golden yellow inside. They do not need pre-soaking, and cook quickly. Mung beans absorb the flavors of spices and seasonings well, possibly the reason why Indians make a curried dish with them to be eaten with steamed rice or bread. Mung beans also lend themselves well to sprouting, and the sprouts are among the most popular ones served in salads, soups, and stir-fries in Asian restaurants and homes.

Nutritional Profile

Like their peers, mung beans are high in protein and fiber, and low in fat, with none of it being saturated. The beans are also quite high in potassium, magnesium, and the B vitamins. When eaten in sprouted form, the nutritional value of the beans becomes even greater, as more of the micronutrients are released in this form.

■ ADZUKI BEANS

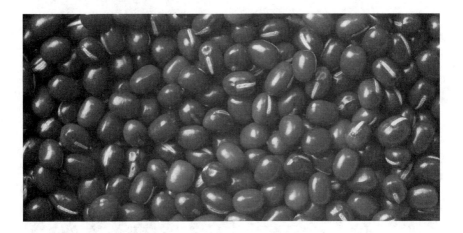

Adzuki beans, also referred to as adukis, or simply as red beans, are an annual vine, with the botanical name *Phaseolus angularis*. Archeological evidence indicates they were first cultivated in Japan between 4000 BC and 2000 BC. Commercial cultivation of these beans in the western hemisphere is fairly recent, the seeds having been brought here from Japan in the early 1970s. While they are eaten in many countries across Asia, they are particularly popular in Japan and China. In Japan, they are the second most important dry beans after soybeans. In China, they are known as *shozu*, meaning *small bean;* its counterpart large bean being the soybean, which is twice as big. The burgundy-red color of the beans is associated with luck and happiness in China. Once skinned and cooked, they have a sweet, nutty flavor and a velvety texture, and this is the reason they are primarily used to make sweets.

Nutritional Profile

Adzuki beans are a good source of protein and soluble dietary fiber, which is regarded as being heart-healthy, and they also contain several vitamins and minerals. A 100 grams serving of cooked adzuki beans offers 128 calories, 0 grams of fat, 7.5 grams of protein, 25 grams of carbohydrates, 7.3 grams of dietary fiber, and only 8 milligrams of sodium. A serving of these beans also provides several vitamins and minerals in amounts equaling significant proportions of recommended daily values—folic acid (30 percent), potassium (15 percent), phosphorus (17 percent), magnesium (13 percent), iron (11 percent), manganese (28 percent), and zinc (12 percent).

■ BLACK-EYED PEAS

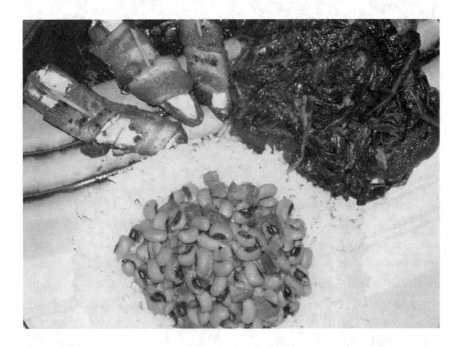

By earliest records in 1674, black-eyed peas originated in West Africa and were brought to the United States with the slave trade. As the climate in the American South is similar to Sub-Saharan

Africa, the crops flourished here. Originally used as food for livestock, the beans became a staple of the slaves' diet. Before arriving in America, these legumes took root in many parts of the world, including many regions of Asia where they are known to grow wild. The name comes from their characteristic appearance, cream-colored oblong beans with a small black dot in the center of the curved inner side resembling an eye. Although called peas, black-eyed peas are actually beans, and are part of the family of beans and peas *Leguminosae* or *Fabaceae*. These attractive, delicious beans are well known in the Southern and Southwestern United States—in fact, few foods are as strongly connected with the Southern culture in the U.S. as black-eyed peas. They even earned a place in history during the Civil War. Black-eyed peas, known also as field peas or cowpeas because they were fed to livestock, were left behind in the fields by Sherman's troops and became an important food for the Confederate South. Eating black-eyed peas and greens on New Year's Day is a tradition in the Southern and Eastern parts of the United States and is believed to bring good luck in the year to come. It is believed that the nearly round peas symbolize coins and the greens symbolize paper money, and the combination, as shown in the figure on the previous page, represents prosperity.

Nutritional Profile

Black-eyed peas are high in protein and soluble fiber, and exceptionally low in calories. When served with a complementary food like rice or corn, they become a complete protein. Although black-eyed peas are plant food, they are included in the *Meat and Beans* category on the Food Guide Pyramid created by the United States Department of Agriculture because they can be used as a protein source, instead of an animal food like meat, at far less cost. The soluble fiber helps lower cholesterol by binding to it and carrying it out of the circulatory system. Black-eyed peas are an especially rich source of potassium, one serving ($1/2$ cup cooked) providing nearly 30 percent of the daily values.

■ CHICKPEAS—GARBANZO BEANS

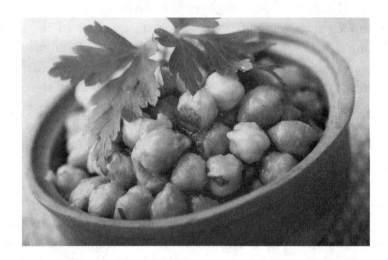

Chickpeas are legumes of the family *Fabaceae,* and Turkey is said to be the center of origin for *cicer,* which has come to be known in the English-speaking world as the chickpea. This legume is known by many other names, including *erébinthos* in classical Greek, *hommes* or *hamaz* in the Middle East, *garbanzo* in Spanish, *ceci* in Italian, *grao-de-bico* in Portuguese, and *kabuli-chana* (to be differentiated from its smaller, darker variety) in India.

Chickpeas are light tan in color when raw, and golden brown when cooked, and they have a thick outer coating, which some recommend removing after soaking and before cooking, for easier digestion. However, researchers have determined that many of the antioxidants present in chickpeas are especially concentrated in the outer seed coat, which makes a case for leaving the skin intact. Chickpeas are sold in many forms—raw dried, canned (cooked), or as flour. At present, chickpeas are grown in the Mediterranean region, Western Asia, the Indian subcontinent, and Australia.

Nutritional Profile

Chickpeas are excellent sources of fiber, folic acid, and manganese. They contain almost twice as much protein as cereal grains, as well as minerals such as iron, magnesium, copper, and zinc. Chickpeas are excellent sources of the essential trace element molybdenum, which is responsible for many biochemical processes at the cellular level. The main nutritional benefits of chickpeas lie in their high-fiber content, antioxidant properties, and lean-protein content. Because the fiber in chickpeas is 65–70-percent insoluble, it remains undigested and takes longer to empty from the stomach, making you feel full and satiated for a long period. This helps control blood sugar, an important health benefit for everyone, but especially for those with adult-onset diabetes or at risk for it. Studies have shown that garbanzo-bean fiber can be metabolized by bacteria in the colon to produce relatively large amounts of certain kinds of fatty acids (SCFAs), which provide energy to the cells that line the intestinal wall. The chickpea fibers can thus help maintain colon health and lower the risk of colon problems.

■ SPLIT PEAS

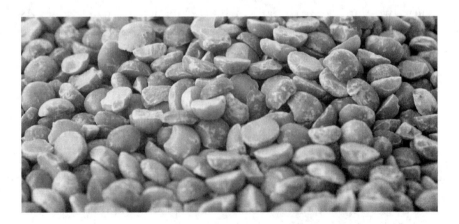

Split peas are a variety of dried peas, which come as either whole or split. Dried peas have been a staple of the human diet since prehistoric times, and for centuries the dry form was the main way people consumed peas. It was not until cultivation techniques created the more tender varieties of garden peas in the sixteenth century that people began to consume peas in their fresh state—it seems the Chinese were the first to consume both the seeds and the pods as a vegetable.

Peas have been found in archeological excavations in Egypt, Asia, and Rome, and they were introduced into United States soon after the colonists first settled in this country. Today, the largest commercial producers of dried peas are Russia, France, China, and Denmark.

Peas belong to the same family as beans and lentils, but are usually distinguished as a separate group because of how they are prepared and because their round shape sets them apart from beans and lentils. Dried peas are the result of harvesting the pea pods when they are fully mature and drying them. Once they are dried and the skins are removed, they split naturally. These peas are usually deep green in color, but they can also be yellow, and either variety can be used interchangeably for most recipes. Unlike fresh peas, dried peas can be enjoyed at any time, for they are available all year.

Nutritional Profile

Split peas are full of fiber—a single cup of cooked dried peas provides nearly two-thirds (65 percent) of the recommended daily value. As previously outlined, soluble fiber forms a gel-like substance in the digestive tract that binds bile (which contains cholesterol) and carries it out of the body. Research has shown that insoluble fiber not only helps to increase stool bulk and prevent constipation, but it also helps prevent irritable bowel syndrome, diverticulosis, and similar digestive disorders. Even more importantly, eating high-fiber foods like cooked peas can prevent weight gain because they take longer to empty out of the stomach, therefore curbing or delaying hunger by keeping you feeling full longer. This also translates into the very significant health benefit of stabilizing blood-sugar levels by preventing them from rising rapidly after a meal. Rapidly rising blood-sugar levels trigger a chain reaction in the body, increasing the risk for adult-onset diabetes over time. In addition, split peas contain significant amounts of protein, the vitamins thiamin and folic acid, and several important minerals. Isoflavones, the phytonutrients contained in the peas, act like weak estrogens in the body, and eating them on a regular basis has been linked to a reduced risk for certain types of cancers, including the breast and prostate cancers.

■ PEANUTS

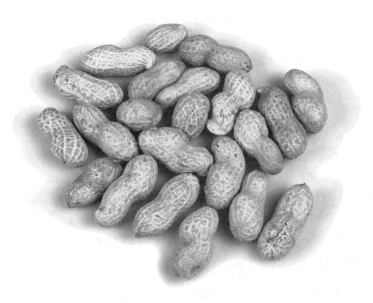

Although believed to be nuts, and eaten as such, peanuts belong to the legume family, *Arachis hypogaea.* The Spanish and Portuguese introduced peanuts to Asia and Africa, and African slaves brought them to North America. Unlike any other legumes, once the flower is fertilized, the peanut plant buries itself in the soil, and the pod develops underground, which is why peanuts are called groundnuts in many parts of the world.

Peanuts are a cash crop in the U.S., where nearly a tenth of the world's supply is grown, half of them in Georgia. About half the peanuts grown in the U.S. are made into peanut butter, a staple in the American pantry—Americans consume 700 million pounds of peanut butter a year. The number of kernels in a pod can vary from two or three to as many as five or seven. There are several varieties of peanuts grown around the world. In the U.S., the Virginia peanut is the one most often eaten whole, in the shell, as *ballpark peanuts,* or as green or boiled peanuts the way they do in the American South. Spanish peanuts, also known as Valencia peanuts, with a red skin and a rich taste, are better known in Europe, but are also used in the U.S. for making peanut butter, peanut oil, and candy bars.

Nutritional Profile

Peanuts are very nutritious, containing 20–30-percent plant protein and 40–50 percent oil, which gives them their rich taste. Because of the high protein and fat content, peanut paste is used to treat malnutrition among infants and children in poorer regions of the world. In clinical studies, peanuts have shown an LDL-lowering (the bad cholesterol) property that is beneficial to heart health. Besides being a rich source of plant protein, peanuts are rich in fiber, vitamins, and minerals, including calcium, magnesium, and potassium, as well as phytochemicals, such as resveratrol (as in red wine) and arginine. At least a quarter of the peanuts produced in the U.S. are eaten as snacks, and they are regarded as a healthy snack.

■ LENTILS

Lentils are believed to have originated and been consumed in central Asia since prehistoric times. Lentil seeds have been unearthed at archeological sites in the Middle East that dated back 8,000 years. Lentils were mentioned in the Bible as the item Jacob traded to Esau for his birthright, and as part of the bread that was made during the Babylonian captivity of the Jewish people. Before the first century AD, they were introduced into India, a country where all legumes, including lentils, are regularly consumed in some form as part of every meal. In many Catholic countries, lentils have long been used as a staple food during Lent. Today, this ancient crop has gained popularity as a versatile legume in both developing and developed countries, and is currently cultivated in more than thirty-five countries, with India, Turkey, Canada, China, and Syria, being the leading commercial producers of lentils.

The botanical name for lentils is *lens ensculenta*. Lentils grow in pods that contain either one or two seeds. There are several varieties of lentils that differ in size, shape, color, consistency, and taste. Different regions and countries around the world have their favorites.

Brown or Green Lentils

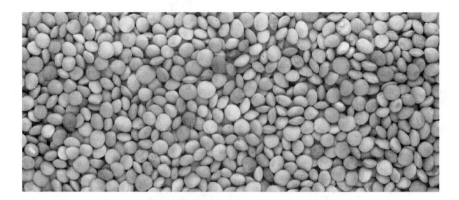

Brown or green lentils, also referred to as Indian brown lentils, German, or continental lentils, and Egyptian lentils, are the ones most frequently eaten in the United States, and the ones you see on grocery shelves everywhere. They tend to get mushy if overcooked, and are therefore best suited for making lentil soup, stews, and casseroles.

French Green Lentils

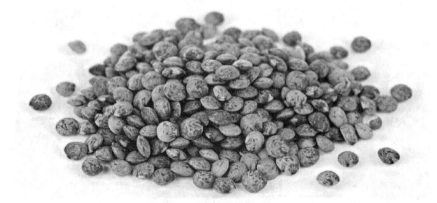

The French call them *lentilles vertes du Puy*, originally grown in the volcanic soils of Puy in France, but now grown in North America and Italy as well. They have a stronger structure than brown or green lentils and tend to hold their shape better when cooked, so they work well in chilled salads or chili.

Red Lentils

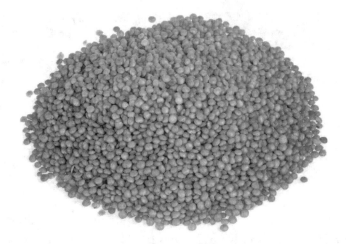

Red lentils are thinner and more fragile, so they tend to break down quickly in the cooking process and become soft and mushy, making them better suited for soups, stews, and casseroles. French green lentils and red lentils may not be as widely available as traditional brown lentils, but if they can be found, their distinct flavor makes them a tasty addition to a variety of dishes.

Beluga Lentils

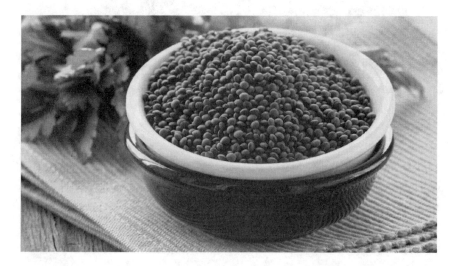

Beluga lentils, also referred to as beluga black lentils and petite beluga lentils, are so named because they glisten like beluga caviar when they're cooked, and this, coupled with their small size, makes them resemble caviar. They're great in soups or salads.

Nearly all the lentil varieties are small relative to the size of peas and beans. They come as round, oval, or heart-shaped disks, yielding varying consistencies when cooked—some become soft and mushy, while others remain firm and whole. The French green, red, or beluga lentils retain their shape better after cooking than the brown or green varieties. The flavor also differs slightly among the varieties, but all lentils share a hearty, dense, and somewhat nutty flavor, and are similar in nutritional value.

Nutritional Profile

The tiny lentils are powerhouses when it comes to their nutritional value, with generous amounts of several healthy nutrients, yet they are low in saturated fat and calories. A standard serving size of any type of lentils is about one quarter cup, which becomes approximately one cup of soft lentils when cooked. On average, one cup of cooked lentils contains 7 grams of fiber, 13 grams of protein, 1 gram of fat, 28 grams of carbohydrates, and 170 calories. The French green lentils are lower in carbohydrates (18 grams vs. 28 grams) and fat (0 grams vs. 1 gram) and therefore lower in calories, containing only 110 calories, no fat, 4 grams of fiber, and 9 grams of protein. When lentils are consumed as sprouts, they generally outperform the cooked ones nutritionally. Fresh, crunchy sprouts have 7 grams of dietary fiber and less than half the calories and carbohydrates of the cooked ones. Compared to cooked lentils and other sprouts, such as alfalfa and radish, sprouted lentils are also significantly higher in protein, iron, and vitamin C. Cooked lentils are, however, higher in some B vitamins, especially folic acid, and in all-important dietary fiber. It is therefore advisable to alternate cooked lentils with lentil sprouts in meals.

Regardless of minor differences in nutrient content, all lentils are high in healthy nutrients like protein, fiber, and vitamins, and low in unhealthy nutrients like fat, particularly saturated fat (essentially absent in lentils). As protein-rich plant foods, lentils are also satiating, and keep you full longer than foods rich in carbohydrates, which helps to prevent weight gain as well as maintain normal blood-sugar levels without extreme fluctuations.

❧ 6 ❧

Cooking, Sprouting, and Storing Legumes

PREPARING LEGUMES FOR COOKING

Harvested crops, like grains, dry beans, peas, and lentils often contain small pieces of rock, dirt, and debris that need to be picked clean. This can be done far in advance of cooking, as, for example, when they are first brought home from the store. The picking can be made into a family activity, children included. Besides being fun, the occasion can be a teachable moment for a lesson on legumes. After picking, the legumes should be stored in dry, airtight containers until ready to be cooked.

If they do not come out of a can, dry beans and peas need to be soaked for several hours prior to cooking (canned beans and peas are, most often, pre-cooked). You can significantly reduce the soaking time by bringing dry beans and peas to a quick boil, draining them, and then adding fresh water to let them soak. An added benefit of this quick-boil-and-drain method is that it cuts down on the potential flatulence of the beans and peas. You also don't need to soak the beans and peas for as long if you use a pressure cooker, and pressure-cooking also cuts cooking time to about one quarter of the traditional method. It's good to remember that dried beans absorb a large amount of water, and the pressure cooker should be no more than one-third full of beans to allow them to expand in the cooker. Microwave cooking is not recommended for dry beans and peas, other than to reheat already cooked or canned ones.

Lentils and split peas do not need soaking. After being picked over and thoroughly rinsed, these are ready for cooking. In cooking, they double in bulk, so they need twice as much water (or broth if you prefer) as other legumes. They take about 20–40 minutes to cook, depending on the variety and age of the legume. Generally, the longer they are stored, the longer they take to cook. Pressure-cooking is not recommended for lentils and split peas, as these legumes tend to get mushy in cooking and may clog the safety valve and cause it to explode, a safety hazard best avoided.

When cooking beans, using the right kind and amount of water is critical. It pays to use soft water, especially if you live in an area where the water has a high mineral content that makes the water hard. You can also get around this by adding a small amount of baking soda (one-eigth teaspoon to a pound of beans) to the water to neutralize the acid. Beans are prone to fermentation, so unless this is your intent, beans should not be allowed to remain at hot temperatures, or even room temperature, for long periods of time. If making a big batch, the leftover beans should be chilled rapidly by placing the pot in a basin of cold water and then refrigerating or storing them in the freezer immediately after cooling. This is especially important in hot, humid weather. The traditional method of cooking beans in Italy, Spain, Greece, and other Mediterranean countries, is to blanch them, bring them to a boil, cook them for five minutes, and then drain and rinse them in cold water. This is believed to preserve the color and texture of the beans. After blanching, beans can be made into any desired dish. Several Asian and African countries routinely ferment their beans to make their culturally unique dishes. If you've ever had the classic South Indian delicacy *dosa*, a thin, crispy crepe stuffed with vegetables, it is made from a mixture of fermented lentil and rice flour. In these regions, fermentation is believed to improve the digestibility of the beans.

All legumes take well to seasonings, such as garlic, onion, parsley, oregano, cilantro, and other herbs. These can be added to the pot at the beginning, or while the legumes are cooking, and their flavors get absorbed into the very permeable skins. Be aware, however, that salt, sugar, molasses, vinegar, and tomatoes harden the skin of the legumes and prevent them from softening, so make sure the legumes are at least halfway cooked and their skins have softened before adding any of these to the dish. Salting is best done just before removing the legumes from heat. If you're pressure-cooking the beans and peas, it's best to salt them before cooking, to keep them from becoming mushy. Frequent stirring of the legumes after they have softened causes them to break up and become mushy, so keep the stirring to a minimum after the beans have softened; instead, resort to shaking the pot or tossing the beans for mixing and turning.

COMBATING FLATULENCE FROM LEGUMES

Intestinal gas is a byproduct of carbohydrate digestion in beans. Since the body lacks the enzyme to digest the *oligosaccharides* naturally found in all seeds, including beans, they pass through the upper digestive tract to the lower intestines mostly undigested. They are broken down by bacteria present in the gut and in the process produce the telltale gas. Given that legumes have been a part of the human diet throughout the ages, people in every region in the world have learned their own unique way of minimizing this problem of flatulence. Some of these are incorporated into the methods of soaking and cooking the beans, others are added to the beans in cooking, and yet others, like the Beano that contains the enzyme needed to digest beans, are taken in pill or liquid form before or with the meal. In India it is customary to eat a piece of crystallized ginger, or chew fennel seeds or betel nuts after every meal to aid in digestion and minimize gas.

In her book on beans, Aliza Green has several tips to combat flatulence from eating beans.[1] First she recommends buying the most recent crop of dried beans and peas because the older they are, the harder it is to digest them. Second, she emphasizes the importance of soaking the beans for several hours, and changing the water at least once during the soaking. Green believes the offending oligosaccharides leach into the water and draining the water gets rid of at least some of them. If doing a quick soak, bring the beans to a boil, cook for 5 minutes, remove from heat, and let soak for 1 hour to achieve the same results. If using canned beans, thoroughly rinse them to remove excess salt as well as some of the sugars. Removing skins from the beans, split peas, and lentils also reduces the amount of gas emitted during digestion. Another tip of hers is to do what people in the Mediterranean do—cook the beans with alkaline-rich greens, such as spinach or chard, to balance the acidity of the beans. Her final recommendation is to cook the legumes in earthenware as is done in Italy, Spain, Greece, Mexico, and Tunisia. Clay is believed to absorb sugars, the offending elements of the beans.

Adding small amounts of ginger, turmeric, fennel, carom seeds, and asafetida (dried plant resin) to beans and lentils during cooking, as people in India do, is also known to keep the flatulence at bay. If all else fails, there are commercial products, like Beano, that contain the enzyme *alphagalactosidase*. These tablets can be taken before eating a meal with beans, or, if in a liquid form, you can take a few drops with the first bite to aid in digestion and keep the gas from forming.

SPROUTING LEGUMES

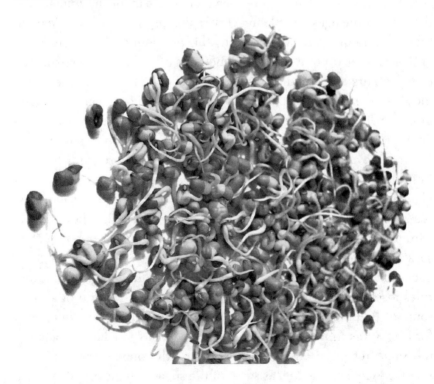

Sprouts are the young shoots of a plant, but not all sprouts are edible. During germination, plants release generous amounts of antioxidants. Bean sprouts pack a punch as a nutritious food, even surpassing the parent seed in micronutrient content. Sprouted legumes are also more easily digested for they have the enzyme that converts carbohydrates into simple sugars. Legumes such as soy and mung beans lend themselves better to sprouting than other beans, and seeds like alfalfa are also sprouted and are highly, famously, nutritious.

Bean sprouts can be purchased commercially, most often in Asian grocery stores. You can also sprout legumes organically at home. Some describe sprouts as a garden in a jar. All you need is a large glass jar, cheesecloth to cover, tepid water, and a rubber band. Rinse thoroughly the beans you want to sprout, place them in a bowl, pour water over them until they are completely immersed, and soak them overnight. In the morning, drain and rinse the beans a few times, changing the water between rinses, then place the beans in the jar, cover it with cheesecloth, and secure it with a rubber band. Add just enough water to cover the beans, without filling the jar to the brim. Turn the jar on it side to spread the beans over a larger area, and place it in a dark, cool (about 70 degrees) place like a closet or pantry. Sunlight or bright light will dry out the beans, warm temperatures might give rise to mold, and too cool temperatures will prevent sprouting. Rinse the beans in the jar by inverting it 1–2 times a day, until the sprouts are fully developed—this may take 3–5 days, or longer for some beans. When the sprouts are about 1" long, rinse them in cold water to remove the seed coats, roots, and other residue, before eating. Bean sprouts are highly nutritious and crunchy, and make a great addition to salads, soups, and sandwiches. The U.S. Food and Drug Administration (FDA) recommends cooking the sprouts before eating to minimize any risk from contaminated sprouts. Cooking them at high temperatures, however, destroys some micronutrients, including vitamin C.

STORING LEGUMES

Legumes can be purchased in bulk and cost significantly less than when buying them in containers. Health food stores often sell them from bins, or you can order them directly from merchants selling dry beans, peas, and lentils and have them shipped to you. They can even be purchased online if stores near you do not carry them. Legumes store well for long periods of time, but need to be stored in dry, air-tight containers at room temperature. They are best when used no later than one year from the date of purchase. After that, they begin to dry out and take much longer to soak and cook. Once cooked, beans can be refrigerated for up to 3–5 days, and stored up to six months in the freezer.

❧ 7 ❧

Recipes

In this chapter, sample recipes are provided for each of the legumes described in Chapter 5. It is best to use dry, raw beans and peas for these recipes, but if canned ones are used, be sure to rinse them thoroughly under running water to remove excess salt and other preservatives added in canning. Follow the tips provided in Chapter 6 for preparing, soaking, and cooking beans and peas. The quick boil-and-soak method (see Table 7.1 below) is recommended for raw beans and peas to cut down on cooking time and minimize the flatulence effect. All lentils, and some beans and peas do not need soaking, including fresh-shelled lima beans, split fava beans, split yellow and red peas, and black-eyed peas. Since all legumes absorb the flavors of seasonings and any other foods with which they are cooked, be sure to make liberal use of your favorite herbs and spices when cooking them. And you might try combining other foods with the legumes.

Many of the recipes provided here have been passed on from one generation to the next in my family. In some cases, they are a variation of the original recipe I developed to incorporate locally available ingredients. All recipes not otherwise attributed come from my family's recipes.

Additionally, you can find an extensive array of recipes for legumes, ranging from simple, easy, and quick to prepare, to very elaborate and fancy dishes in cookbooks dedicated to legumes, such as *Beans* by Aliza Green.[1] And you can also find recipes for legumes on popular cooking websites, such as allrecipes.com, foodnetwork.com, savvy vegetarian.com, jamieoliver.com, and lentilworld.com.

The Indian and Indian-inspired recipes included here call for spices commonly used in that cuisine. These are often sold as curry powder. You can also make this blend in small quantities at home and store it in airtight jars for reuse. A recipe for homemade curry powder is given here.

Homemade Curry Powder

MAKES 3 OUNCES

$1/4$ cup coriander seeds

2 tablespoons cumin seeds

2 dried red chili pods,
slit in the middle and seeded

$1/2$ teaspoon whole cloves

4 cardamom pods, skins removed and discarded

1 teaspoon ground cinnamon

1 teaspoon ground turmeric

1. Place a small, dry frying pan over low heat; add all the ingredients, except the ground cinnamon (if using) and turmeric; lightly dry roast until the fragrances of spices are released, but not smoking. Remove from heat; add the ground cinnamon and turmeric to the pan. Let the mixture cool.

2. Transfer the mixture of spices to a spice mill (or a pestle and mortar) and grind to a powder. Store in an airtight jar.

SLOW-SOAK AND QUICK-SOAK METHODS
FOR DRIED BEANS AND PEAS

DRIED BEANS/PEAS	SLOW-SOAK METHOD	QUICK-SOAK METHOD
Red kidney, pinto, black beans, cannellini, and navy beans	Soak 6 hours at room temperature; if using a pressure cooker, soak in lightly salted water so skins stay intact under pressure.	Bring to a boil and cook 2 minutes; remove from heat and soak 1 hour at room temperature.
Fava beans (brown), Large lima beans	Soak 12 hours at room temperature; in hot, humid weather, change water once to prevent fermentation.	Bring to a boil and cook 5 minutes; remove from heat and soak 1 hour at room temperature.
Whole chickpeas	Soak 10 hours at room temperature; in hot, humid weather, change water once to prevent fermentation.	Add a pinch of baking soda to water, bring to a boil, and cook 3 minutes; remove from heat and soak 1 hour at room temperature.
Mung beans, adzuki beans	Soak 8 hours at room temperature.	Bring to a boil and cook 1 minute; remove from heat and let soak 1 hour.

Red Kidney Beans

The kidney bean, also known as the red, or chili, bean, is generally considered the bean of choice when preparing *chili con carne* (chili pepper with meat). Countless local variations of this famous spicy dish can be found all over the world, as well as in many American Tex-Mex and fast-food restaurants. Red kidney beans are used in New Orleans and much of southern Louisiana for the classic Creole dish of red beans and rice. Louisiana families, particularly those with a recent Caribbean heritage, use the smaller, darker red beans, and a smaller variety of these kidney beans is also used in the La Rioja region of Spain, in a popular, distinguished local dish called *caparrones*.

In the northern region of India, red kidney beans, called *rajama* in Hindi, are prepared as *dal*, a generic curried dish eaten regularly with flat bread, known locally as *chapatti*, that resembles the Mexican tortilla. These beans are especially good in simmered dishes where they absorb all the flavors of the seasonings and foods with which they are cooked. Many other ideas for enjoying kidney beans can be found in recipe books and cooking websites.

Curried Red Kidney Beans (Rajma Dal)

This is a popular way for Indians to enjoy these meaty legumes.

SERVES 4

2 cups dry kidney beans

1 large onion, chopped

4 cloves garlic, chopped

2-inch piece fresh ginger, peeled and chopped

1 hot green chili pepper, slit, seeded, and chopped

4 tablespoons vegetable oil

1 teaspoon ground cumin*

1 teaspoon ground turmeric*

$1/2$ teaspoon ground red chili pepper*

$1/2$ teaspoon ground cinnamon*

$1/2$ teaspoon ground cloves*

2 teaspoons ground coriander*

1 cup chopped tomatoes

Salt to taste

1 teaspoon granulated white or brown sugar

1 tablespoon chopped fresh cilantro

These spices are sold as a blend (curry powder) in grocery stores and online. Check label for ingredients listed, and if any of the above are missing from the list, add them separately in cooking.

1. Rinse and soak the beans (consult the table on methods at the beginning of the chapter for soak time). Drain water, rinse thoroughly, and set aside. If using canned beans, skip this step, but thoroughly rinse beans under running water to remove excess salt.

2. Grind the chopped onion, garlic, ginger, and chili pepper into a paste.

3. Heat the oil on medium heat, add the paste, ground cumin, turmeric, ground red chili, cinnamon, cloves, and coriander, and cook for 2–3 minutes, stirring frequently to prevent the mixture from sticking to the bottom of the pot. Drain off the excess oil, add beans and enough water to cover the beans. Cook for one hour or until the beans are tender and smash easily between the fingers; check frequently and add water if necessary. About halfway through cooking, add the tomatoes, salt, and sugar.

4. Remove from heat after the beans are completely cooked, and garnish with fresh, chopped cilantro leaves.

Serve with freshly cooked white or brown rice, or warm *chapattis.*

Authentic Louisiana Red Beans and Rice

SERVES 8

$1/4$ cup olive oil

1 large onion, chopped

1 green bell pepper, chopped

2 tablespoons minced garlic

2 stalks celery, chopped

1 pound dry kidney beans, rinsed and soaked using the quick-soak
or soaked overnight for at least six hours

10 cups water

2 bay leaves

$1/2$ teaspoon cayenne pepper

1 teaspoon dried thyme

$1/4$ teaspoon dried sage

1 tablespoon dried parsley

1 teaspoon Cajun seasoning

1 pound Andouille sausage,* sliced

2 cups long grain white rice

For a vegetarian version, replace sausage with sliced Portobello mushrooms.

1. In a skillet, heat oil over medium heat. Cook onion, bell pepper, garlic, and celery in olive oil for 3 to 4 minutes.

2. Rinse beans and transfer to a large pot with 6 cups water. Stir cooked vegetables into beans. Season with bay leaves, cayenne pepper, thyme, sage, parsley, and Cajun seasoning. Bring to a boil, and then reduce heat to medium-low. Simmer for $2^{1}/_{2}$ hours.

3. Stir sausage into beans, and continue to simmer for 30 minutes.

4. Meanwhile, prepare the rice. In a saucepan, bring 4 cups of water and rice to a boil. Reduce heat, cover, and simmer for 20 minutes.

Serve beans over steamed white rice.

Recipe provided by Allrecipes.com. Recipe submitted by Miami Beach at Allrecipes.com.

Spicy Turkey Chili

*This dish can be a little too spicy for some.
If less heat is desired, omit the habanero pepper,
or reduce the amount of chili powder.*

SERVES 8

2 tablespoons olive oil

1 onion, chopped

5 cloves garlic, minced

2 small green bell peppers, seeded and chopped

1 habanero pepper, seeded and chopped

2 pounds lean ground turkey*

2 tablespoons chili powder

2 teaspoons red pepper flakes

1 tablespoon paprika

1 tablespoon ground cumin

2 teaspoons dried oregano

1 teaspoon ground black pepper

1 (1-ounce) envelope instant hot chocolate mix

2 teaspoons seasoned salt

1 tablespoon Worcestershire sauce

1 teaspoon liquid smoke flavoring

2 (14.5-ounce) cans diced tomatoes
with green chili peppers, drained

1 (8-ounce) can tomato sauce

1 (15-ounce) can kidney beans, drained

$1/3$ cup beer (optional)

$1/2$ cup canned whole-kernel corn

1 tablespoon hot pepper sauce

*For a vegetarian version, replace turkey meat with diced vegetables.
Bell peppers, carrots, celery, and zucchini work well.*

1. Heat the olive oil in a large saucepan over medium heat. Add the onion, garlic, green peppers, and habanero pepper; cook and stir until the onion is transparent. Push these to one side of the pot, and crumble in the ground turkey. Cover, and cook for about 5 minutes, stirring occasionally, or until the meat is no longer pink. Stir everything together so the garlic doesn't burn.

2. Season with chili powder, red pepper flakes, paprika, cumin, oregano, black pepper, hot cocoa mix, and seasoned salt. Stir in Worcestershire sauce, liquid smoke, diced tomatoes with green chilies, tomato sauce, and the beans. Pour in the beer, if using. Partially cover the pan, and simmer for about 50 minutes, occasionally stirring the pot carefully, so as to not break up the beans.

3. Mix in the corn and hot pepper sauce, and simmer for 10 more minutes. Remove from the heat, and let it cool for a few minutes before serving.

Recipe provided by Allrecipes.com. Recipe submitted by Corwyn Darkholme at Allrecipes.com.

Pinto Beans

Pinto beans are eaten in the United States and Northwestern Mexico as whole beans in broth or mashed and refried. In the mashed or refried form, they are a customary filling for burritos and many other dishes in Tex-Mex restaurants. In addition to kidney beans and black beans, pinto beans are often used in the preparation of *chili con carne*. Rice and pinto beans served with cornbread or corn tortillas are often a staple meal in Mexico when meat is unavailable or unaffordable. In Brazil, pinto beans, called by their local Portuguese name *feijão carioca*, are regularly accompanied by rice, potatoes, or yams. In Spain, a red variety of the pinto bean, known as *pinta alavesa*, is quite popular in the Basque region of Northern Spain, where it originated. Here, in October, the locals celebrate a pinto bean fair called the *Feria de la alubia pinta alavesa*. Other pinto-bean varieties that are consumed around the world include the Burke, Maverick, Othello, and Sierra.

Slow-Cooker Pinto Beans

The beans in this easy recipe turn out perfectly,
without even a single bean left uncooked or partially cooked.

SERVES 8

1 pound dried pinto beans, rinsed and quick-soaked
or soaked overnight;

1 onion, chopped

$3/4$ green bell pepper, diced

2 celery ribs, chopped

3 cloves garlic, chopped

1 pound ham, cubed

1 teaspoon ground cumin, or to taste

1 tablespoon dried oregano, or to taste

2 bay leaves

1 tablespoon lard*

5 cups chicken broth, or as needed to cover the beans

For a healthier version, use 1 tablespoon of olive oil instead.

1. Rinse and drain the soaked pinto beans and put in a slow cooker.

2. Place onion, green bell pepper, celery, garlic, ham, cumin, oregano, bay leaves, and lard (or olive oil) in slow cooker.

3. Pour enough chicken broth into the slow cooker to cover the other ingredients.

4. Cook on low until beans are very tender, 5–6 hours.

Top with your favorite garnishes and serve with warm rice or whole-wheat tortillas.

Recipe provided by Allrecipes.com. Recipe submitted by Corena at Allrecipes.com.

Pinto Beans and Yellow Rice

*This popular Puerto Rican dish can also be made with
red kidney or black beans. This recipe is a contribution
from the in-law side of my family.*

SERVES 6

6 cups water

1 (6-ounce) can tomato sauce

2 cups uncooked rice, rinsed, drained, and set aside

8 tablespoons vegetable oil or olive oil divided into 2 equal parts

1 large onion, coarsely chopped

6 cloves garlic, peeled

1/2 green bell pepper, coarsely chopped

1/4 cup chopped cilantro, divided into two equal parts

12 ounces dry pinto beans, rinsed, and quick soaked

2 teaspoons fresh oregano, finely chopped

1 tablespoon parsley, chopped

1 bay leaf

1 packet achiote (sold in Hispanic aisle of grocery stores)

1 teaspoon vinegar

1 lemon, juiced

1/2 teaspoon lemon zest

1 teaspoon fresh cracked pepper

1 teaspoon salt or to taste

1. In a food processor or blender, mix the chopped onion, garlic, bell pepper, half of the chopped cilantro, and half the oil. Grind to a coarse paste. This is referred to as *sofrito* in Puerto Rican cooking.

2. Give the quick-soaked beans a final rinse and place them in a large, heavy-bottomed pot. Pour the water over the beans, making sure they are completely submerged, adding more water if necessary. Stir in the bay leaf, half of the *sofrito,* and the lemon zest; cover the pot and bring to a boil.

3. Lower the heat and simmer for 1 hour or until the beans are soft, but not mushy. Test by holding a bean between the thumb and index finger—

the bean should be soft to the touch, but should have retained its shape. Stir in the lemon juice, vinegar, and all of the herbs; sprinkle with salt, and pepper. Remove from heat, sprinkle the remaining chopped cilantro on the dish, and set aside.

Instructions for yellow rice

1. Add the remaining oil to a pot over medium heat. When the oil is hot, but not smoking, add the remaining sofrito paste and the packet of achiote powder (to give the rice the golden yellow color), and cook for 2 minutes; add the rice and sauté for 2 minutes, frequently stirring to keep the rice from sticking to the bottom of the pot. Add tomato sauce and $2^1/_2$ cups of water.

2. Bring to a boil, lower the heat, cover and simmer until the rice is cooked, about 35–40 minutes. Stir frequently to make sure the rice is cooked evenly and is not sticking to the bottom of the pot.

Serve the rice warm with the pinto beans. If desired, you can complement this rice-and-bean meal with chicken or other meat.

Black Beans

The black bean and its close relative the black turtle bean are not only nutritional superstars, but also lend themselves to a broad variety of recipes, from salads and soups to main dishes, snacks, and relishes. Black beans are very popular in Brazil, Cuba, Mexico, Trinidad, and the American Southwest. Since these beans are notorious for causing the offending flatulence, to minimize gas production in the gut, it is especially important to use the quick-boil-and-soak method when using the raw, dry beans. In various areas of Brazil, it is a very regularly consumed bean, the main ingredient in their national dish, *feijoda,* and also a main ingredient of *Morosy Cristianos* in Cuba. It is a must-have in the typical *gallo pinto* of Costa Rica and Nicaragua, and is a fundamental part of *pabellón criollo* in Venezuela. This bean is found in the Cajun and Creole cuisines of South Louisiana, and in such Mexican-American dishes as the black bean burrito.

Black turtle beans are very popular for making soups. In one form or another, they are served in almost all of Latin America, as well as in many Hispanic enclaves in the United States. It is a normal practice to save the boiled water of these beans, which acquires a black coloring, and consume it, with seasonings, as a soup, known as *sopa negra* (black soup). Further, it is used as broth in dishes, including *caldo de frijol* (bean broth), and is used in small quantities to season or color *gallo pinto* or other dishes.

Quinoa and Black Beans

This recipe combines a star legume and a star grain. The dish is a more nutritious and flavorful alternative to rice and black beans, and can be eaten as a meal with or without meat.

SERVES 10

1 onion, chopped

3 cloves garlic, peeled and chopped

$3/4$ cups uncooked quinoa

$1/2$ cups vegetable broth

1 teaspoon ground cumin

$1/4$ teaspoon cayenne pepper

Salt and pepper to taste

1 cup frozen corn kernels

2 (15-ounce) cans black beans, rinsed and drained

$1/2$ cup chopped fresh cilantro

1. Heat the oil in a saucepan over medium heat. Stir in the onion and garlic and sauté until lightly browned.

2. Mix quinoa into the saucepan and cover with vegetable broth. Season with cumin, cayenne pepper, salt, and pepper. Bring the mixture to a boil. Cover, reduce heat, and simmer 20 minutes.

3. Stir frozen corn into the saucepan, and continue to simmer for about 5 minutes until heated through. Mix in the black beans and cilantro.

Serve warm with a salad on the side.

Recipe provided by Allrecipes.com. Recipe submitted by 3LionCubs at Allrecipes.com.

Southwest Black Bean Chicken Soup

*This slow-cooker recipe is as easy and flavorful
as it is healthy.*

SERVES 8

1 pound cooked dark-meat chicken

3 (15.5-ounce) cans black beans,
drained and rinsed

2 (14-ounce) cans chicken broth

2 (10-ounce) cans diced tomatoes
with green chili peppers

1 (15.25-ounce) can whole kernel corn

$1/2$ large onion, chopped

$1/2$ cup chopped jalapeño peppers

2 cloves garlic, chopped

$2^1/_2$ teaspoons chili powder

2 teaspoons red pepper flakes

2 teaspoons ground cumin

1 teaspoon ground coriander

Salt and freshly ground black pepper to taste

$1/2$ cup sour cream*

Use the fat-free kind for a healthier version.

1. Place the chicken, black beans, chicken broth, tomatoes with green chili peppers, corn, onion, jalapeño peppers, garlic, chili powder, red pepper flakes, cumin, coriander, salt, and black pepper in a slow cooker.

2. Cook on low for 8 hours.

Add about a tablespoon sour cream on each serving, and serve with warm corn bread or rice.

Recipe provided by Allrecipes.com. Recipe submitted by Beth at Allrecipes.com.

Cuban Black Bean Soup with Smoked Turkey

SERVES 8

2 cups black turtle beans, soaked (use the
quick-boil-and-soak method), drained, and rinsed

1 medium onion, peeled

8 garlic cloves, peeled

3 bay leaves

2 quarts low-sodium chicken stock

2 quarts cold water

2 tablespoons peanut or other vegetable oil

1 large white or yellow onion, diced

1 tablespoon minced garlic

1 tablespoon ground cumin,
lightly toasted in a dry pan

1 tablespoon paprika

1 packet of achiote seasoning*

1 pound smoked turkey legs

1 can plum tomatoes, chopped

2 tablespoons malt or sherry vinegar

Salt and pepper to taste

*Available in grocery stores in the Latin food aisle. This seasoning is made from annatto
seed oil. The oil is extracted from the seeds and filtered for use in cooking to add a rich
orange-yellow color and a mild flavor. The process is labor-intensive, and although the die-
hard Cuban and Puerto Rican cooks do it for their special occasion dishes, the commercially
available substitute in the powder form serves the purpose, and is recommended.

1. Place the soaked beans in a large pot, along with the whole onion,
garlic cloves, bay leaves, and the turkey legs. Cover with chicken stock
and cool water. Bring to a boil, skim off any foam that rises to the surface, and reduce heat to a simmer. Cook for about 2 hours (or 25–30 minutes in a pressure cooker, starting the timer after the steam has built up
in the cooker), or until the beans are soft. Remove and discard the onion,
garlic cloves, and bay leaves. When the turkey legs are cool enough to
handle, strip the meat from the bone, dice, and reserve.

2. Purée three-fourths of the beans, along with their liquid, in a blender or food processor. Leave the remaining cooked beans whole. Strain the puréed beans through a sieve to remove the skins. Return them to the pot along with the remaining whole beans.

3. In a skillet, heat the oil. Add the diced onion, minced garlic, cumin, paprika, the contents of the achiote packet, and the reserved diced turkey meat. Sauté until the mixture softens. Add the tomatoes and vinegar, stirring the mix. Add this mix to the pot with the beans, and bring the soup to a boil. Season to taste with salt and pepper.

Serve with sliced avocado or other garnishes of your choice.

Cannellini Beans

Cannellini beans have a slightly nutty taste and mild earthiness, and their thin skin allows them to absorb flavors well. The absorbability of flavors and the ability to retain their shape in cooking make this bean very versatile. They are among the best white beans for salads and ragouts.

Tuscan White Bean Stew

SERVES 6

2 cups dried cannellini or other white beans,
picked over, rinsed, soaked overnight, and drained

6 cups water

1 teaspoon salt

1 bay leaf

2 tablespoons olive oil

1 yellow onion, coarsely chopped

3 carrots, peeled and coarsely chopped

6 cloves garlic, chopped

$1/4$ teaspoon freshly ground black pepper

1 tablespoon chopped fresh rosemary, plus 6 sprigs

$1/2$ cups vegetable stock or broth

1. In a soup pot over high heat, combine the white beans, water, $1/2$ teaspoon of the salt, and the bay leaf. Bring to a boil over high heat. Reduce the heat to low, cover partially, and simmer until the beans are tender, 60 to 75 minutes. Drain the beans, reserving $1/2$ cup of the cooking liquid. Discard the bay leaf. Place the cooked beans into a large bowl and save the cooking pot for later use.

2. In a small bowl, combine the reserved cooking liquid and $1/2$ cup of the cooked beans. Mash with a fork to form a paste. Stir the bean paste into the cooked beans. Return the cooking pot to the stovetop and add the olive oil. Heat over medium-high heat. Stir in the onion and carrots and sauté until the carrots are tender-crisp, 6–7 minutes. Stir in the garlic and cook until softened, about 1 minute. Stir in the remaining $1/2$ teaspoon salt, pepper, chopped rosemary, bean mixture and stock. Bring to a boil, and then reduce the heat to low and simmer until the stew is heated through, about 5 minutes.

Ingredients for croutons

1 tablespoon extra-virgin olive oil

2 cloves garlic, quartered

1 slice wholegrain bread, cut into $1/2$-inch cubes

Instructions for croutons

1. To make the croutons, heat the olive oil over medium heat in a large frying pan. Add the garlic and sauté for 1 minute. Remove from the heat and let stand for 10 minutes to infuse the garlic flavor into the oil. Remove the garlic pieces and discard. Return the pan to medium heat. Add the bread cubes and sauté, stirring frequently, until lightly browned, 3–5 minutes. Transfer to a small bowl and set aside.

To serve, ladle stew into warmed bowls and sprinkle with the croutons. Garnish each bowl with a rosemary sprig and serve immediately.

Recipe reprinted courtesy of Mayoclinic.com.

Cannellini Bean and Vegetable Soup

SERVES 6

1 tablespoon butter

1 tablespoon olive oil

4 leek bulbs, chopped

1 medium onion, chopped

2 potatoes, peeled and diced

4 cloves garlic, minced

1 teaspoon ground cumin

1 green chili (serrano or jalapeño) pepper, deseeded and finely chopped

3 carrots, peeled and diced

2 celery stalks, leaves removed and sliced

3 cups low-sodium vegetable broth

2 cups water

1 cup white wine (optional)

$1/2$ teaspoon chopped fresh rosemary

$1/2$ teaspoon chopped fresh sage

1 (15-ounce) can cannellini beans, rinsed and drained

1 cup fresh or frozen and thawed spinach, chopped

Salt and black pepper to taste

1. Heat the butter and olive oil in a large heavy-bottomed soup pot over medium heat. Add the leeks and onion, and cook until softened and translucent, about 4 minutes. Add the potatoes and sauté for 3–4 minutes, giving them a head start, as they take longer to cook than other vegetables. When the potatoes are halfway cooked, stir in the garlic, cumin, chili pepper, and all vegetables except the spinach. Continue cooking until the vegetables are almost, but not quite, done.

2. Add the broth, water, and white wine (if using) to the pot. Stir in rosemary and sage. Bring to a boil, then reduce heat to low. Add the cannellini beans, spinach, salt, and black pepper, and simmer, covered, for 20 minutes more, or until the potatoes are soft to touch.

Serve warm with a crostini or a slice of toasted whole wheat bread.

Mexican Bean Salad

The beauty of this salad recipe is that it calls for three different legumes, making it into a true powerhouse, nutritionally speaking.

SERVES 6–8

1 (15-ounce) can cannellini beans, drained and rinsed

1 (15-ounce) can black beans, drained and rinsed

1 (15-ounce) can kidney beans, drained and rinsed

1 green bell pepper, chopped

1 red bell pepper, chopped

1 (10-ounce) package frozen corn kernels

1 red onion, chopped

$1/2$ cup olive oil

$1/2$ cup red wine vinegar

2 tablespoons fresh lime juice

1 tablespoon lemon juice

2 tablespoons white sugar

1 tablespoon salt

1 clove crushed garlic

$1/4$ cup chopped fresh cilantro
(reserve a few whole stems to garnish prior to chopping)

$1/2$ tablespoon ground cumin

$1/2$ tablespoon ground black pepper

1 dash hot pepper sauce

$1/2$ teaspoon chili powder

1. In a large bowl, combine beans, bell peppers, frozen corn, and red onion.

2. In a small bowl, whisk together olive oil, red wine vinegar, lime juice, lemon juice, sugar, salt, garlic, cilantro, cumin, and black pepper. Season to taste with hot sauce and chili powder

3. Pour olive oil dressing over vegetables; mix well. Chill thoroughly.

Garnish with reserved cilantro leaves and serve cold.

Recipe provided byAllrecipes.com. Recipe submitted by Karen Castle at Allrecipes.com.

Tuscan Chard and Cannellini Bean Soup

This is a hearty soup that does not take much time to make.
The soup thickens as it stands due to the pasta and the cheese in it.

SERVES 6

2 slices smoked bacon, finely chopped

1 onion, chopped

1 clove garlic, minced

$1/4$ teaspoon freshly grated nutmeg (optional)

1/8 teaspoon crushed red pepper flakes (optional)

6 cups chicken broth, or more as needed

1 (15-ounce) can cannellini beans, drained and rinsed—or more to taste

2 tablespoons chopped sun-dried tomatoes

2 ounces Parmesan cheese rind

1 bunch red, white, or rainbow Swiss chard

$1/4$ cup uncooked small pasta, such as orzo or pastina

5 large fresh sage leaves, minced

5 leaves fresh basil, coarsely chopped (optional)

1 tablespoon grated Parmesan cheese, divided (optional)

1 tablespoon extra-virgin olive oil, divided (optional)

1. In a large saucepan over medium heat, cook the bacon, onion, garlic, nutmeg, and red pepper flakes until the onion is translucent, about 5 minutes. Pour in chicken broth and cannellini beans, and bring the mixture to a boil. Stir in sun-dried tomatoes and the piece of Parmesan cheese rind. Reduce heat to a simmer, and cook while you prepare the chard, about 10 minutes.

2. Cut the stems from the chard, and slice the stems into pieces about $3/4$-inch long. Cut the chard leaves into 1-inch wide ribbons. Stir the chard stems and pasta into the soup, setting aside the leaves. Reduce heat to a simmer, and gently simmer until the pasta is tender, about 10 minutes. Stir the chard leaves, sage, and basil into the soup, and simmer just until wilted, 3–4 minutes.

Ladle soup into bowls and serve topped with Parmesan cheese and a drizzle of olive oil, if desired.

Recipe provided by Allrecipes.com. Recipe submitted by Callinectes Sapidus at Allrecipes.com.

White (Navy) Beans

Also known as Boston beans, white coco, or pea beans, navy beans are used for baked beans, purées, soups, and stews. This is the bean used in the well-liked baked beans of New England, as well as in various soups, such as the Senate bean soup. The bean is also used in some pies. Dry navy beans are available year-round in pre-packaged containers as well as bulk bins. Canned navy beans are also widely available at local markets and grocery stores.

Boston Baked Beans

SERVES 6

2 cups navy beans

$1/_2$ pound bacon*

1 onion, finely diced

3 tablespoons molasses

$1/_4$ teaspoon ground black pepper

$1/_4$ teaspoon dry mustard

$1/_2$ cup ketchup

1 tablespoon Worcestershire sauce

$1/_4$ cup brown sugar

For a healthier option, use turkey bacon.

1. Soak beans, using the quick-soak method or overnight in cold water. Simmer the beans in the same water until tender, approximately 1–2 hours. Drain and reserve the liquid.

2. Preheat oven to 325°F (165°C). Arrange the beans in a 2-quart bean pot or casserole dish by placing a portion of the beans in the bottom of dish, and layering them with bacon and onion.

3. In a saucepan, combine molasses, pepper, dry mustard, ketchup, Worcestershire sauce, and brown sugar. Bring the mixture to a boil and

pour over the beans. Pour in just enough of the reserved bean water to cover the beans. Cover the dish with a lid or aluminum foil.

4. Bake for 3–4 hours in the preheated oven, until beans are tender. Remove the lid about halfway through cooking, and add more liquid if necessary to prevent the beans from getting too dry.

Serve warm with freshly baked bread or other cooked grains.

Recipe provided by Allrecipes.com. Recipe submitted by Ajrhodes3 at Allrecipes.com.

Fava Beans/Broad Beans

Although fava beans have long been a staple in Asia, the Middle East, and parts of Latin America, North Africa, and Europe, until fairly recently they have remained little known and consumed in the U.S. This was despite the fact they were first introduced in North America in 1602, and found their way to Virginia by 1648 and New England by 1671. The lack of enthusiasm for fava beans in the past may be due to the fact that Americans have never developed a taste for bitterness. Here, bitter is bad, sweet is good, whereas, in many cuisines, the two are considered equally desirable, not negative and positive.

More Americans are discovering the buttery texture and lovely nutty taste of the fava bean. During the season, fresh fava beans in the pod are sold in farmers' markets and in the produce section of many grocery stores. Fava beans are prepared and consumed in many different ways around the world, excluding the one cited in the famous quote of Anthony Hopkins in the movie *Silence of the Lambs*. In Rome, on the first of May, Roman families traditionally eat fresh fava beans with Pecorino Romano cheese. In Southern Italy, the beans are puréed with wild chicory to make a popular Puglian dish. In Central Italian regions, a once popular food, the Bagiana, has been recently rediscovered as a fancy food. It is a soup of fresh or dried fava beans, seasoned with onions and beet leaves stir-fried in olive oil and lard before being added to the soup (if trying this dish, you might want to replace the lard with a vegetable oil, for health reasons).

Along the Northern Mediterranean, the dry fava beans are eaten boiled, and sometimes combined with garlic sauce (*skordalia*). In Greece, the bean is called a broad bean because another bean, the yellow split bean, is called the fava bean there. Italians like them in salads and stews, or simmered with tomatoes and sprinkled with grated Pecorino Romano. Spaniards pair the beans with spicy chorizo sausage or salty Serrano ham. In Portugal, a single bean is included in the *Bolo-Rei*, Christmas cake, and the tradition is for the person who gets the slice with the bean to buy the cake the following year.

In Egypt, *ful* is prepared from the small round bean, known as the *ful hammam,* cooked until very soft. The dish is eaten as a staple in Egypt, but it is also popular in the cuisines of Syria, Turkey, and Saudi Arabia. In Syria and Turkey, the dish is served mixed with *tahini* (sesame paste) and olive oil, topped with aleppo pepper (a variety of capsicum) sauce. Eating ful in this manner is also popular in Israel where it was introduced by immigrant Yemenite Jews. In Iran, the beans are cooked with rice to make *Baghalee Popo* in *Farsi* (rice with broad beans), one of the most famous dishes there.

In most Arab countries, the bean is used for a breakfast dish called *ful medame,* with chopped parsley, onion, garlic, and lemon juice. The fava beans are left simmering in large copper jars throughout the night, to be served the next morning.

In China, Thailand, Colombia, and Peru, the beans are fried, causing the skin to split open, and are then salted and spiced to eat as a delicious, crunchy, savory snack. In the Sichuan province of China, a paste called *doubanjiang* is made by combining fermented fava beans and soybeans with salt, rice, and spices. The people of Sichuan refer to this salty, spicy paste as the *soul of Sichuan cuisine* and use it as a flavoring agent for fried tofu dishes and cold tofu salads. A similar form of bean paste called *gochujang* is used in Korean cuisine.

Fava Bean Breakfast Spread

This Egyptian breakfast dish made with dry fava beans has origins that reach back to the time of the pharaohs, and it is still eaten today by many Egyptians.

SERVES 6

I pound dry fava beans*, quick-soaked or soaked overnight (12 hours) or use 2 cans (15 ounces each) for immediate use

2 tablespoons olive oil

1 tablespoon melted butter

1 medium onion, chopped

4 garlic cloves, finely chopped

1 teaspoon cumin

$1/_8$ teaspoon cayenne pepper

$1/_2$ cup red lentils, rinsed and drained

1 cup water

1 cup chopped tomatoes

2 tablespoons lemon juice

Salt to taste

*The smaller variety of fava called ful hammam is used by Egyptians in this dish. The larger fava, called ful rumi, is the kind found more often in American markets, and it can be used instead.

1. Rinse and drain the beans. Place the favas in a large pot and add enough fresh water to cover the beans by 2 inches. Bring to a boil, reduce heat to very low, cover and simmer for 8 hours, skimming the froth off the top occasionally. If using the canned favas, skip the boiling and the long simmering. Simply rinse and set aside.

2. Heat the oil and butter over medium heat; Add the onion and cook until it softens and turns translucent; Add the garlic, cumin, cayenne pepper and cook for 1 more minute; Add the lentils and water; cook until the lentils are soft, about 15 minutes. Add the fava beans and chopped tomatoes and cook for 5 more minutes.

3. Remove from heat and lightly mash the cooked beans and lentils together with a potato masher or a thick wooden spoon. Stir in the lemon juice and salt.

Serve with pita bread, and hard-boiled eggs (optional).

Recipe provided by Allrecipes.com. Recipe submitted by Beverly Estes at Allrecipes.com.

Falafel with Fava Beans and Chickpeas

Falafel can be made with either fava beans or chickpeas, but using the combination yields a better texture and taste to the dish. The ingredients used in this dish are similar to those used in an Indian dish, which made an adaptation of this recipe possible.

SERVES 8

$1/2$ cups dried, shelled (skinless) fava beans,
quick-soaked or soaked overnight in cold water,
water changed once to prevent fermenting

$1/3$ cup dry chickpeas quick-soaked or soaked
in cold water for 10 hours, changing water once
to prevent fermentation in hot humid weather

1 yellow onion, finely chopped

$1/4$ cup parsley leaves, minced

$1/4$ cup cilantro leaves, minced

2 garlic cloves, minced

1 teaspoon ground cumin

1 teaspoon baking powder

1 teaspoon salt

$1/2$ teaspoon ground coriander

$1/4$ teaspoon cayenne pepper (or less for less heat)

Vegetable oil, for frying

Tahini sauce, for serving, and pita bread (optional)

1. After draining and rinsing both the fava beans and the chickpeas, place them in the bowl of a food processor, along with the onion, parsley, cilantro, garlic, cumin, baking powder, salt, ground coriander, and cayenne. Pulse the mix until a coarse paste is formed. Add a small amount of water, if needed, to make the paste hold together—adding too much water makes the mixture too thin and unsuitable for making patties or balls. Check the batter for consistency by pressing the mixture together between the fingers. Remove the mixture to a bowl and set aside for about 30 minutes. In hot weather, keep it refrigerated.

2. In a saucepan (or deep-fryer preheated to 350°F), pour enough vegetable oil so it is standing at least 3" above the base. Scoop the fava/chickpea mixture into $1^{1}/_{2}$–2-tablespoon increments and shape into balls or patties about $1^{1}/_{2}$–2 inches in diameter. Gently lower them into the hot oil, making sure they don't fall apart. Fry the falafel in batches until crisp and brown on all sides, turning to promote even browning, 2–$2^{1}/_{2}$ minutes. Transfer to paper-lined plates to blot excess oil. Serve with tahini sauce and pita bread (optional).

INGREDIENTS FOR TAHINI SAUCE

1 cup tahini paste (available in stores)

Juice of 2 lemons

$1/_{2}$ teaspoon minced garlic

Salt

Instructions for Tahini Sauce

Tahini sauce can be prepared by combining the tahini paste with the lemon juice and salt to taste. Any leftover sauce must be refrigerated.

Lima Beans

Shelled lima beans (the pod is not edible) are available fresh or frozen, canned, or in dry form. Dry lima beans need to be boiled until tender. They can be served by themselves (dressed with vinaigrette) or may be added to soups and stews to infuse flavor. Lima beans contain hydrogen-cyanide gas in low levels that gets neutralized in cooking, and this is why lima beans should not be eaten raw. Because of the ease with which this bean can be stored as provisions on ships and transported, explorers and merchants favored lima beans for their crews. Lima beans are now cultivated around the world.

Lima Beans with Roasted Eggplant

Indians incorporate eggplant in a variety of dishes, much like the Mediterraneans. Roasted and mashed eggplant is combined with sweet peas in a dish called baingan barta. I substitute lima beans for peas as they are meatier and retain their shape better.

SERVES 6

1 large eggplant, whole

$1/4$ cup peanut oil or other vegetable oil

1 teaspoon mustard seeds (optional)

1 medium onion, chopped

5 cloves garlic, finely chopped

1" piece fresh ginger, minced

$1/2$ teaspoons ground cumin

$1/2$ teaspoon ground turmeric

1 fresh green chili, seeded and finely chopped

1 package (10 ounces) frozen lima beans, thawed

1 large tomato, chopped

$1/2$ teaspoon salt, or to taste

2 tablespoons chopped fresh cilantro (coriander)

1. Preheat the oven to 400° for 10 minutes. Rinse and dry the eggplant. Smear about a tablespoon of the oil on the eggplant, making sure the entire skin of the eggplant is covered. Using a fork, punch a few holes in the skin of the eggplant so it won't burst open in the oven. Place the eggplant in an ovenproof dish and roast it in the pre-heated oven for 25 minutes. Remove from the oven and let it cool. Peel the skin off the eggplant, which should come off easily. Slit it in the middle, and using a spoon or fork, remove as many of the seeds as possible, and discard. Mash the seeded eggplant, and set aside.

2. Heat the remaining oil in a skillet over medium heat. Add the mustard seeds (if using), and cover with a sputter guard. Fry for 30 seconds, and add chopped onion and cook till onions soften, for about 2 minutes. Stir in the garlic, ginger, cumin, turmeric, and chili pepper. Cook for 2 more minutes. Lower the heat and add the lima beans and chopped tomatoes. Cook for 8–10 minutes or until the lima beans are tender to touch.

3. Stir in the reserved eggplant, salt, and all but a teaspoon (to be used as garnish later) of the chopped cilantro. Cook the mixture for another 5 minutes on low heat. Remove from heat, garnish with the reserved cilantro.

Serve warm with rice or whole-wheat chapatti (or tortilla).

Golden Risotto with Baby Lima Beans and Red Pepper

SERVES 4

1 large pinch of saffron threads

$1/2$ cup dry white vermouth (or any dry white wine)

$3^1/2$ cups vegetable stock or chicken stock

2 tablespoons unsalted butter

$1/2$ cup onion, chopped

2 tablespoons shallots, chopped

1 red bell pepper, seeded and diced

1 teaspoon garlic, chopped

1 cup raw Arborio or other short-grain rice

1 package (10 ounces) frozen baby lima beans

$1/4$ cup freshly grated Parmigiano-Reggiano cheese

2 tablespoons Italian parsley leaves, chopped

1. Add the saffron threads to the dry white vermouth (or dry white wine) and reserve.

2. Pour the stock into a saucepan and bring to a simmer over medium heat, reduce the heat, and keep it simmering.

3. In a second large saucepan over medium heat, melt the butter. Add the onion, shallots, red pepper and cook, stirring frequently, for 5 minutes, or until the onion is soft. Stir in the garlic and rice. Cook 2 minutes, stirring constantly. Stir in the reserved vermouth-saffron mixture and bring to a boil. When the vermouth has been absorbed, add $1^{1}/4$ cups of the simmering stock. Bring to a boil, reduce the heat, simmer uncovered, stirring occasionally, until most of the liquid is absorbed. Stir in another $1^{1}/4$ cups of the simmering stock and the lima beans. Simmer uncovered, stirring occasionally, until most of the liquid is absorbed. Stir in the remaining cup of stock and continue cooking until the liquid has been absorbed and the rice is tender, about 15 minutes. Stir in the cheese and parsley, and season to taste with salt and black pepper.

Serve warm with a salad on the side.

Reprinted from Beans *by Aliza Green. Available from Running Press, an imprint of The Perseus Books Group. © Copyright 2004.*

Soybeans

Japanese use soybeans in making *tamari*, a sauce that is thicker than the regularly encountered soy sauce, but similar in taste, and *miso*, a fermented soybean paste used as a flavoring agent. Other fermented soybean foods include the all-familiar soy sauce, *natto*, and *tempeh*. Many people have also eaten edamame, boiled or steamed, green, crunchy pods that are served before meals at Japanese restaurants and bars. They are a fresh form of soybeans and are as delicious as they are nutritious. Dry soybeans are used in making a curd, known by its Japanese name, tofu, that is sold in Asian markets, and large grocery chain stores in metropolitan areas in the U.S. While tofu is bland in taste, it absorbs flavors well and can be transformed into tasty dishes with the addition of herbs and spices. Soybeans in different forms are frequently added to other foods during processing. Soybean oil, a vegetable oil low in saturated fats, is ordinarily used in Chinese cooking for its mild taste and flavor-infusing property.

Edamame (Green Soybeans) with Garlic

This crunchy, delicious, and fun snack is often served in Japanese restaurants, to be enjoyed while you wait for your food. The following recipe is my homemade version. It is a low-calorie substitute for snacks and appetizers made with bread and other fatty ingredients.

SERVES 4

6 cups of water

1 pound frozen edamame (green soybeans in the pod, found in the frozen vegetable section of Asian stores and many large grocery stores)

1 tablespoon vegetable oil

8 cloves garlic, finely chopped or minced

1 teaspoon oyster sauce or light soy sauce

$1/2$ teaspoon white pepper

$1/4$ teaspoon cayenne pepper

1. Fill a heavy-bottom pot two-thirds with water, and bring to a boil. Add the frozen edamame from the bag, and cook for 35–40 minutes or until the beans are tender in the pod. Remove from heat and set aside.

2. Heat the oil in a skillet over medium heat. Add the garlic, and cook for 1 minute or until the garlic turns slightly brown, add the oyster (or soy) sauce, stir, and remove from the heat immediately. Add the reserved edamame and mix well to coat them with the sauce.

Place the edamame in a serving bowl, sprinkle with the white and cayenne peppers, and serve with a glass of wine or sake (optional).

Mung Beans

Mung beans are incorporated extensively in the cuisines of Asia, including India, Pakistan, Sri Lanka, China, Japan, Thailand, Taiwan, Vietnam, and Korea. In India, *Mung Dal,* a soupy dish made with mung beans, is very popular, and is eaten with steamed rice or home-made bread. Here they also use the flour of mung beans to make a savory crepe enjoyed with peanut or coconut chutney. In neighboring China, mung-bean flour is used to make sweets like *tangshui,* a particularly popular one that is served warm or cold.

In China, starch is also extracted from mung beans to make jellies and transparent, or cellophane, noodles. In Indonesia, mung beans are used to make a popular dessert snack called *Es Kacang Hijau* that has the consistency of porridge. In the Philippines, they are the main ingredient of the dessert *Hopiang Munggo.* Here, mung beans are also used to make a savory dish called *Ginisang Monggo* with chicken or pork, shrimp or fish. When made with shrimp or fish, it is traditionally served on Friday evenings, as the majority of the Filipino people are Roman Catholic and don't eat meat on Fridays. Mung-bean sprouts are used in stir-fry dishes in several regions of Southeast Asia.

Saucy Mung Beans
(Indian Mung Dal)

SERVES 6

1 cup dry split mung beans
(split mung beans come skinless and cook fast).

3 cups water

1 tablespoon melted butter or vegetable oil

1 teaspoon mustard seeds
(sold in Indian grocery stores, and online)

1 teaspoon cumin seeds

4 cloves garlic, coarsely chopped

3 twigs fresh curry leaves
(sold in Indian and Chinese grocery stores;
they add a rich flavor to the dish; if unavailable
use 2 tablespoons chopped cilantro leaves instead)

$1/2$ teaspoon turmeric

$1/2$ teaspoon cayenne pepper

$1/2$ teaspoon ground cumin

1 onion, finely chopped

1-inch piece fresh ginger, minced (optional)

1–2 jalapeños or other hot green chilies, halved,
seeded, and finely chopped

1 fresh tomato, diced

1 teaspoon salt, or to taste

1. Thoroughly rinse the beans under cold running water, and place in a pot. Cover with water so the beans are completely submerged, and soak for 1 hour. Drain and rinse the beans and set aside. Place 3 cups of water in a pot and bring it to a boil. Add the beans and cook for 30 minutes or until the beans are soft and mushy. Remove from heat and set aside.

2. Heat the butter or oil in a large saucepan over medium heat. Add the mustard, cumin seeds, garlic, and curry leaves, and sauté for a minute or two. Be careful, as the seeds will splatter in the hot oil, so it is a good idea to use a splatter guard. Next add the ground spices, stir for a few seconds, and then add the onion, minced ginger (if using), and chopped green chilies to the pan. Sauté until the onion begins to brown. Add the diced tomatoes, cover, and cook until the tomatoes are soft and turning saucy.

3. Add the cooked mung beans, and three-quarters of a cup of water (less if thicker sauce is preferred) to the pan. Reduce the heat and simmer for 20 minutes, adding more water if necessary. Add salt to taste, stir in the chopped cilantro (if using in place of curry leaves) near the end of the cooking time, and remove from heat.

Serve hot with fresh cooked rice, chapatti, or nan (Indian flatbreads).

Mung Bean Crepes
(Pesarattu or Dosa)

This dish, often eaten at breakfast or as a snack in the afternoon, was my childhood favorite and continues to be a favorite to this day. It does take some practice to get crepes perfect, but once you master the technique, they come out perfect every time. The crepes are as delicious as they are nutritious, and you are sure to impress your guests with this unusual dish.

SERVES 4 (8 CREPES)

$1/2$ cup whole mung beans with skin

$1/2$ cup uncooked rice

8 teaspoons of peanut or other vegetable oil

2 jalapeño or other hot green chilies, halved, seeded; 1 coarsely chopped, and 1 finely chopped and reserved for topping the crepe

1 small onion, finely chopped

$1/2$-inch fresh ginger, coarsely chopped

1 teaspoon cumin seeds (or $1/2$ teaspoon ground cumin)

2–3 sprigs curry leaves, stripped of the stem and coarsely chopped, reserving one half of the leaves for topping the crepe

$1/4$ cup chopped cilantro

1 teaspoon salt

1 tablespoon butter for additional flavor (optional)

$1/4$ teaspoon *asafetida* (optional) to minimize flatulence; available in Indian grocery stores, and online

1. Cover the raw mung beans with water and soak overnight. This will produce the desired mild fermentation. Next morning, drain the water and rinse thoroughly. If not using immediately, refrigerate, as you do not want the fermentation to continue.

2. Rinse and soak the rice separately in a bowl for 3–4 hours. Drain the water from the rice and set aside.

3. Grind the coarsely chopped ginger, cumin, chilies, and curry leaves in a blender or food processor with a little water. Add the rice, and continue

to add water in small increments until you get a smooth batter. Add the mung beans, and grind until the batter's consistency is such that it is easily spreadable (medium-coarse) on the griddle, adding small amounts of water as needed. Add salt and *asafetida* (optional) to the batter.

4. Heat a flat-iron griddle, and when hot, reduce heat to medium. Have a bowl of cold water ready and sprinkle a spoonful on the hot griddle, to keep the batter from sticking to the griddle (a trick I learned from my mother). Stir the batter and pour a ladleful in the center of the griddle and start spreading outward in circles (like making a pancake). As the crepe starts to cook, drizzle a teaspoon of oil all around it. Once the crepe starts to crisp on the top, flip it. Sprinkle a tablespoon of chopped onion, the finely chopped green chili, curry leaves, and cilantro on the top and let it cook until the crepe is crisp and slightly brown on the edges. Fold the crepe as you would an omelet to keep the toppings from falling out. If desired, spread a small amount of butter on top for flavor and to keep the crepe from drying out. Repeat for each crepe.

Serve the crepes warm with Tomato Chutney (*see* recipe below).

Tomato Chutney

*This chutney is hot and spicy, and needs to be used
sparingly—about 1–2 teaspoons per person.*

4 medium-sized ripe tomatoes

2 dry red chilies, seeded, coarsely chopped

2 jalapeño or other hot green chilies, halved, seeded, and chopped

4 cloves garlic, chopped

1 teaspoon mustard seeds

1 teaspoon cumin seeds

4 teaspoons peanut or other vegetable oil

1 teaspoon chopped coriander (cilantro) leaves

$1/2$ teaspoon sugar

$1/4$ teaspoon turmeric

Salt to taste

1. Heat the oil in a saucepan. When hot, reduce heat and add the mustard and cumin seeds, wait until the seeds start to sputter, add the red chilies and sauté for a few seconds until chilies are brown. Add the chopped garlic, green chilies, and chopped tomatoes. Sauté the mix for 1–2 minutes, until the tomatoes are soft but not mushy. Remove from the heat, wait until the mix cools, and add the salt, sugar, and chopped cilantro. Place the mix in a blender and blend until it reaches a smooth (or medium coarse if desired) paste. It is not necessary to add water, as the tomatoes have plenty of juice in them.

Place the chutney in a serving bowl.

Leftover chutney will last up to a week in the refrigerator.

Mung Bean and Rice Pilaf (Khichidi)

This one-pot meal is often served for breakfast in India to keep school-going children satisfied until lunchtime. It also works well for lunch on a weekend or a light supper when a heavy meal is not desired.

SERVES 6

1 cup split mung beans without the skin

2 cups long or short grain rice, uncooked

1 medium onion, coarsely chopped

2 (fewer if milder heat is preferred) green chili peppers,
seeded and chopped

5 whole cloves

2 sticks of cinnamon

1 bay leaf

1-inch piece of ginger, skinned and minced

1 cup whole green beans, stems removed
and cut into large pieces

1 green bell pepper,
seeded and cut into 1-inch pieces

1 red bell pepper,
seeded and cut into 1-inch pieces

$1/2$ cup sliced mushrooms

$1/4$ cup whole cashew nuts (optional)

$1/2$ teaspoon ground turmeric

1teaspoon ground cumin

2 tablespoons chopped sweet basil

4 tablespoons vegetable oil

2 tablespoons melted butter

4 cups water

1. Rinse mung beans and rice. Soak them together in cold water for 20 minutes. Drain and set aside.

2. Heat the oil and butter together in a large, heavy, pot on medium heat. Lightly fry the cashew nuts (if using) until they turn golden brown, scoop them up with a slotted spoon, and place them on a plate lined with a paper towel. Add the bay leaf, cloves, and cinnamon, and fry for 30 seconds. Add the onion, green chili pepper, and ginger. Cook until the onions turn translucent. Stir in the turmeric, ground cumin, and the cut green beans. Cook for 2–3 minutes until the beans are halfway cooked, then add all the other vegetables. Stir well and cook for another 2 minutes. The vegetables should not be fully cooked at this point.

3. Add the rice and mung beans. Stir well and add salt and water, making sure the water is standing at least 1 inch above the mixture. Bring to a boil, and lower the heat. Cover and simmer for 25 minutes or until the rice and beans are fully cooked, adding small amounts of water along the way, if necessary. A minute before removing from heat, stir in the chopped basil and the cashews.

Serve warm with sliced cucumbers and tomatoes on the side.

Adzuki Beans

In Japan, adzuki beans are boiled, mashed, and combined with sugar and shortening to make a paste used in a variety of sweet dishes, from puddings and ice cream to stuffed pastries and a filling for steamed buns. The majority of Japanese sweets contain adzuki beans in some form. Adzuki-bean ice cream made with Japanese red adzuki beans, ginger, and green tea is quite popular in Japan, and was first served in Chinese and Japanese restaurants to please visiting Americans who wanted something sweet after their meal. Some Asian cultures enjoy red-bean paste as a filling or topping for various kinds of waffles, pastries, baked buns, or biscuits. In Asian stores, adzuki paste is sold in cans. It is also common to add flavoring, such as chestnut, to bean paste and use it as an ingredient in many dishes. Boiled adzuki beans with sugar and a pinch of salt are made into a red-bean soup in China. Adzuki beans are also eaten sprouted or boiled to make a hot tealike drink.

There are ways of utilizing this star legume in savory dishes as well. Here are two examples.

Adzuki Bean Mango Stir-Fry with Cilantro, Lime, and Coconut Sauce

SERVES 4

1 tablespoon peanut oil or other vegetable oil

1 red onion, cut into 1 inch long strips

1 green bell pepper, cut into 1 inch long strips

$1/2$ cup carrots, thinly sliced

1 cup canned adzuki beans, drained and rinsed

2 small mangoes, nearly ripe, but firm, peeled, and cut into strips

1. Heat the oil in a wok or large skillet over medium-high heat. Cook the onion, bell pepper, and carrots in the hot oil until the carrot is tender, about 10 minutes.

2. Add the adzuki beans and mango; cook and stir until the mango is hot.

3. Remove from heat and set aside.

Ingredients for sauce

1 cup light coconut milk

$1/2$ cup fresh cilantro, chopped

1 lime, juiced

1" piece of fresh ginger, peeled and minced

1 clove garlic, minced

1 tablespoon agave nectar (available in specialty grocery stores)

Instructions for sauce

1. Blend the coconut milk, cilantro, lime juice, ginger, garlic, and agave nectar in a blender until smooth.

2. Pour the sauce over the stir-fried vegetables.

Serve over a bed of freshly made rice.

Recipes provided by Allrecipes.com. Recipes submitted by Tori Farbisz at Allrecipes.com.

Adzuki Beans with Baby Bok Choy

The mild-flavored Chinese greens, bok choy, combine well with the slightly sweet-tasting adzuki beans. If bok choy is not available in your area, delicately flavored baby broccoli can be used instead.

SERVES 6

1 cup uncooked fresh adzuki beans or 1 can (15 ounces) cooked

1 tablespoon olive oil

2 cloves garlic, peeled and crushed

$1/2$ pound chopped baby bok choy (or baby broccoli)

2 tablespoons water

$1/4$ cup tamari (Japanese-style soy sauce that is thicker, darker, and stronger in flavor)

1 teaspoon ground cumin

1 teaspoon ground fresh cilantro (coriander)

Salt and pepper to taste

1. If using fresh beans, place them in a medium saucepan with enough water to cover. Bring to a boil, reduce heat, and simmer 30–45 minutes, until the beans are tender. If using canned beans, drain and rinse them thoroughly. Set the beans aside.

2. Heat olive oil in a skillet over medium heat, and sauté garlic about 1 minute. Mix in the chopped greens, and 2 tablespoons water. Season the mix with tamari, ground cumin, and cilantro. Stir in adzuki beans and mix well. Reduce heat to low, cover, and simmer for about 15 minutes, or until the greens are tender. Add salt and pepper, just before the end of cooking.

Serve with freshly cooked white or brown rice.

Black-Eyed Peas

On a trip back from the South one New Year's Day, I happened to stop for lunch during a brief layover at Atlanta airport and had a chance to witness that holiday's Southern tradition of eating black-eyed peas. One of the eateries had an especially long line because, I learned, they were serving black-eyed peas and collard greens as side dishes to their entrées. Eating black-eyed peas is not limited to New Year's Day, however. These tasty legumes are enjoyed throughout the year in many parts of the world. They were popular in Africa, long before being brought to the American South. They are part of African-American soul food and are key to the dish hoppin' John (black-eyed peas, rice, and pork). Black-eyed peas are sold in the market as fresh in the pod, frozen, or dried. The fresh-shelled and frozen forms of the peas don't need to be pre-soaked for cooking, but the dry peas do have to be pre-soaked for several hours, or overnight. Black-eyed peas mix well with other legumes, meat, poultry, spices, and chilies.

Black-Eyed Peas
with Pork and Greens

This recipe is a variation of the dish Hoppin' John. The dish contains three kinds of pork meat and is as scrumptious as can be—certainly a treat to be had on special occasions, like New Year's Day, but not meant to be a regular on your plate.

SERVES 8

1 pound dried black-eyed peas, rinsed and quick-soaked, or soaked overnight

1 pound pork neck bones

3 slices bacon, cut into $1/2$-inch pieces

1 cup diced onion

1 cup diced celery

1 cup diced carrot

3 cloves garlic, chopped

6 cups cold water

1 bay leaf

1 teaspoon dried thyme

$1/2$ teaspoon ground cumin

$1/2$ teaspoon ground black pepper

1 pinch cayenne pepper, or to taste

1 (10-ounce) can diced tomatoes with green chili peppers

1 teaspoon salt

6 ounces smoked ham, diced

1 bunch kale, ribs removed and leaves torn into pieces

1. Drain black-eyed peas and set aside.

2. Cook pork necks and bacon in a Dutch oven over medium heat until lightly browned, about 5 minutes

3. Stir in onion, celery, and carrot; cook and stir until the vegetables are softened, 6–7 minutes. Stir in garlic and cook 1 minute.

4. Pour cold water and black-eyed peas into pork mixture; increase heat to high.

5. Stir in bay leaf, thyme, cumin, black pepper, and cayenne pepper. Bring mixture to a simmer, reduce heat to low, cover and simmer for 45 minutes.

6. Stir in tomatoes and salt. Simmer uncovered until beans are tender, about 40 minutes.

7. Remove neck bones from mixture; separate any meat from bones, return meat to Dutch oven, and discard bones.

8. Stir in diced ham and kale; cook until greens are tender, 10–15 minutes.

Serve over steamed rice, couscous, or quinoa.

Recipe provided by Allrecipes.com. Recipe submitted by Chef John at Allrecipes.com.

Black-Eyed Peas and Baby Kale Salad

SERVES 6

1 cup dried black-eyed peas, or 2 cups frozen

1 head garlic, outer skin removed and 1″ cut off the top
to expose the cloves

1 whole dry red chili pepper pod

2 cups baby kale, triple rinsed and blotted dry

2 tablespoons peanut oil or other vegetable oil

1 cup fresh corn kernels, or 1 package (10 ounces) frozen

1 medium onion, diced

1 red or yellow bell pepper, seeded and diced

$3/4$ cup malt or cider vinaigrette (make your own or purchase)

Salt and pepper to taste

$1/4$ cup candied walnuts

2 tablespoons fresh parsley, chopped

3 or 4 celery ribs, thinly sliced

1. If using dry black-eyed peas, soak them using the quick-soak method (boil for 5 minutes and soak for 1 hour at room temperature), rinse, and place them in a heavy-bottomed pot with 4 cups of cold water, garlic head, and the red pepper pod; bring them to a boil, skimming off and discarding any foam that rises to the surface.

2. Reduce heat and simmer for 1 hour or until the peas are soft. If using frozen black-eyed peas, combine them with 3 cups cold water with the garlic and red pepper pod, bring to a boil and simmer for 30 minutes.

3. After the peas are fully cooked and tender, but not mushy, remove from the heat, then remove and discard the garlic head and the chili pepper pod. Allow the peas to cool in the liquid briefly. Drain off any excess liquid, rinse the peas, and set aside.

4. Place a sauté pan on medium-high heat; add the oil, and sauté the corn until crispy, but tender. Stir in the onion, sliced celery ribs, and diced bell peppers, and cook for 1 minute. Remove the pan from the heat.

5. Place the baby kale loosely at the bottom of a salad bowl and stir in the black-eyed peas and sautéed vegetable-corn mixture. Pour on the vinaigrette and toss gently. Season with salt and pepper, and sprinkle with candied walnuts and chopped parsley.

Serve immediately or store in refrigerator.

Chickpeas (Garbanzos)

If you've ever dined at a Middle Eastern restaurant, you would have been served pita bread with hummus, a purée of chickpeas mixed with lemon juice, garlic, and tahini, a sesame-seed paste. Ground chickpea batter is the main ingredient in the Greek dish falafel. In India, chickpea flour is used to make the Southern dish dosa (a round, thin crepe served plain or stuffed with vegetables), and *pakoras* (vegetable fritters). Chickpea flour is turned into a batter and baked to make *farinata,* a thin, unleavened pancake (crepe) that originated in Italy and later became popular in France. Chickpeas are slowly finding their way into the American diet in different forms. Mature chickpeas are cooked and eaten cold in salads, added to stews, ground into flour, and turned into many different dishes—a standard feature of salad bars is a bowl of raw, presoaked chickpeas ready to be added to a salad.

Tempura-Style Vegetables (Pakoras) with Mint Chutney

This dish is served as an appetizer or a savory snack at teatime in India, and is popular with all ages. You will find it on the menu in Indian restaurants under appetizers.

SERVES 6

2 cups chickpea flour, sold in Indian grocery stores as *besan*, as well as in some large grocery stores

1 teaspoon ground cumin

1 teaspoon cumin seeds

1 teaspoon carom seeds, sold in Indian stores as *ajwain*, and in specialty food stores

$1/4$ teaspoon ground cayenne pepper

1 teaspoon salt

1 teaspoon ground turmeric

$1/2$ cup water

Peanut or other vegetable oil for frying

1 head cauliflower, separated into 2" florets, each sliced into wedges in the middle

1 cup spinach leaves, washed, blotted dry, stems cut off, and kept whole

1 large potato, peeled and sliced into rounds $1/4$-inch thick

1. To make the batter, mix the chickpea flour and all ingredients except the oil and vegetables. Slowly add water to the flour while mixing the batter by hand, adding small amounts of water as needed. Test the consistency by placing a drop of it on a plate with water. The batter should remain nearly intact without spreading. I learned this plate test from my mother.

2. Half fill a frying pan or a fryer with the oil and place it over medium heat. When the oil is hot, test it by dropping a tiny amount of the batter in the oil. If it surfaces quickly, it is ready. One at a time, alternately dip the cauliflower and the potato into the batter and drop slowly into the oil, taking care not to splash the hot oil on your hands. Fry each vegetable 2 minutes, or until it is fried on all sides, turning once with a slotted spoon. Use the spoon to remove the fried pieces to a plate lined with paper towels. Repeat until all the vegetables are fried, doing the spinach leaves last as they take less time to fry. Keep these pakoras warm until the mint chutney is ready.

Ingredients for mint chutney

1 cup fresh mint leaves

$1/2$ cup fresh cilantro, corsely chopped

1 hot green chili pepper, slit, seeded and chopped

1 small onion, coarsely chopped

4 cloves garlic, peeled

1 teasppon ground cumin

2 tablespoons, freshly squeezed lemon juice

1 teaspoon sugar

$1/2$ teaspoon salt

Instructions for mint chutney

1. Place all ingredients in a food processor or blender and grind to a smooth paste, adding small amounts of water, no more than a spoonful at a time to avoid making the paste too watery.

To serve, put the chutney in a small bowl as a dipping condiment for the vegetable *pakoras.* Place it in the center of the table near the vegetables for everyone to serve themselves.

Chickpea Curry (Channa Masala)

This dish is commonly eaten in all regions of India, and seems to have gained popularity with non-Indians as well, for it routinely appears on the menu of Indian restaurants in the U.S and U.K.

SERVES 8

1 pound dried or 2 cans (15 ounces each) chickpeas
(if using dry ones, consult the table on methods at the beginning
of the chapter for soak time; skip this step if using canned beans)

2 tomatoes, diced

1 jalapeño or other green chili pepper, seeded, chopped

1 piece fresh ginger (1 inch), peeled and roughly chopped

4 cloves garlic, chopped

1 onion, chopped

1 tablespoon peanut or other vegetable oil

1 teaspoon ground turmeric

1 teaspoon cumin seeds

1 teaspoon salt or to taste

2 tablespoons *channa masala* (an inexpensive spice blend sold in Indian grocery stores as *channa* or *chhole masala*.)
If you cannot find it, you can also blend it at home by combining the ingredients below:

- 1 tablespoon dry mango powder or dry pomegranate powder
- 1 teaspoon cumin seeds
- 1 teaspoon coriander seeds
- 1 teaspoon fennel seeds
- 1 red chili pepper, seeded

Lightly roast and grind the above together into a coarse blend.

1 teaspoon chopped fresh cilantro for garnish

1. Drain water from the chickpeas, rinse and place in heavy-bottomed pot. Add 6 cups of cold water, and cook over medium heat for 90 minutes or until the peas are tender, but still have their shape intact. Remove from heat and set aside. If using canned chickpeas, drain the juice from the cans completely, rinse them thoroughly, and set aside.

2. Combine the tomatoes, diced chili pepper, ginger, garlic, half the chopped onion, and $1/2$ cup of the cooked chickpeas. Mince into a course paste, and set aside. Place another $1/2$ cup of chickpeas in a bowl, mash them coarsely with a heavy spoon or potato masher, and set aside.

3. Heat the oil in a large skillet over medium-high heat, add the turmeric and cumin seeds, and cook for a few seconds or until the cumin seeds swell and turn golden brown. Add the remaining onion and cook for about 3 minutes or until the onion is translucent. Stir in the blended tomato mixture, the mashed and whole chickpeas, the channa masala blend, salt, and 1 cup of water (less if thicker consistency is preferred). Cover and cook for 10–15 minutes or until you can easily mash a chickpea between two fingers. Remove from heat, and garnish with the chopped cilantro.

Serve with freshly made basmati rice (fragrant, long grain rice) or chapatti (Indian flat bread).

Hummus

*After eating store-bought hummus for many years,
I started making my own. It certainly proved worth the
effort because it tastes fresher and more flavorful
without the added preservatives.*

SERVES 12

3 garlic cloves, finely chopped or minced

2 15-ounce cans of garbanzo beans (chickpeas),
drained and rinsed

2/3 cup of tahini paste (available in specialty stores
or large grocery stores

$1/3$ cup freshly squeezed lemon juice

$1/2$ cup water

$1/4$ cup olive oil

$1/2$ teaspoon of salt

Pine nuts (toasted) as needed

1 tablespoon chopped parsley for garnish

1. In a food processor, combine the garlic, garbanzo beans, tahini, lemon juice, $1/2$ cup water, and olive oil. Mince and blend to a smooth paste, adding small amounts of water if necessary. Add salt to taste.

2. Spoon into serving dish and sprinkle with toasted pine nuts and chopped parsley.

Serve with raw dip vegetables, such as carrots or celery, or pita chips (toasted pita bread).

Instructions for pita chips

Cut pita bread into thin triangles, brush with olive oil, and toast for 10 minutes in a 400°F oven. Or you can purchase pita chips in specialty stores.

Split Peas

The standard way that Americans eat split peas is in split pea soup, either with pieces of ham or pork added, or kept vegetarian with no meat added. A bowl of this thick, hearty, and tasty soup can be a meal in itself, or it can be eaten as a starter. If you think only one kind of soup can be made with split peas, get wowed by the number and variety of recipes and serving suggestions for this soup offered by Split peaSoups.com, a website devoted solely to this purpose.

This legume is also eaten in other ways across the globe. In Morocco, a soup made with split peas and pumpkin is regarded as golden by the Jews there, and is served traditionally on the first night of Rosh Hashanah, the Jewish New Year. In India, the peas are cooked into a soupy dish called dal, and eaten with rice or bread as part of a meal. Split peas are also ground into flour in India, and the batter is used to make tempura-style vegetable fritters.

Moroccan Split Pea and Pumpkin Soup

SERVES 8

3 quarts chicken stock
(or vegetable broth for a vegetarian version)

1 quart cold water

1 pound (2 cups) dried yellow split peas,
rinsed and drained

3 bay leaves

1/3 cup olive oil

2 large onions, chopped

1 tablespoon ground fresh ginger

1 tablespoon ground cinnamon

2–3 pinches of saffron threads, crumbled

2 pounds peeled and diced red pumpkin,
butternut squash, or calabaza

Salt and freshly ground black pepper

1. In a large soup pot, combine the chicken stock (or vegetable broth), water, yellow split peas, and bay leaves, and bring to a boil on medium-high heat. Skim off and discard any foam that forms on the surface. Reduce the heat and simmer for about 30 minutes, or until the split peas become tender.

2. Heat the olive oil in a skillet over medium heat and add the onion, ginger, cinnamon, and saffron. Cook until the onions are softened, but not browned. Add this mixture and the pumpkin cubes to the soup in the pot. Simmer for 30 more minutes, or until the pumpkin is quite soft. Remove from heat, and discard the bay leaves. Season to taste with salt and pepper.

Serve the soup hot.

Recipe reprinted from Beans *by Aliza Green. Available from Running Press, an imprint of The Perseus Books Group. Copyright © 2004.*

Peanuts

Ask any child in the U.S. what their favorite food is, and you are bound to hear a peanut butter and jelly sandwich mentioned, possibly more often than any other food. As well, roasted peanuts are sold as a snack food everywhere, from ballparks to movie theaters, and they are routinely served on airplanes. Many Asian recipes incorporate peanuts and peanut products, such as crumbled peanuts, ground peanut paste, and peanut oil, into their dishes. Thai appetizers, for example, are served with a spicy peanut sauce, and in India, several breakfast foods are served with a *chutney* made of ground peanuts and coconut.

Three-Legume Snack

I was inspired by the commonly sold mixed nuts to come up with a snack that combines several legumes in a snack. The result was this three-legume combination snack. Although one of the ingredients in the recipe is deep-fried, it beats the widely consumed potato chips and other high-fat, empty-calorie snack foods in taste and flavor as well as nutritional value.

SERVES 10

1 pound dry-roasted peanuts, without the shell

1 cup dry, large, split golden fava beans, quick-soaked, drained and rinsed, blotted dry in a clean cloth or layers of paper towels, at least 2 hours before use

1 cup whole mung beans with the skin, rinsed and soaked in cold water for 30 minutes, drained and blotted dry in a clean cloth or layers of paper towels, at least 2 hours before use

$1/2$ teaspoon sea salt

1 teaspoon ground cayenne pepper

1 teaspoon garlic powder (optional)

2 tablespoons coarsely chopped curry leaves, or

1 tablespoon dry mint leaves

Peanut or other vegetable oil for frying

1. Half fill a deep pan or fryer with oil and heat over medium heat. Fry the mung beans until crisp and remove with a slotted spoon to a plate lined with paper towels. The skins may become loose, but do not remove them, as they add nutritional value as well as taste and color.

2. Add the chopped curry leaves to the hot oil remaining in the pan (if using dry mint leaves, skip this step as they do not need frying), and fry for 30 seconds. Remove the leaves with a slotted spoon, and place them next to the already fried beans.

3. Preheat the oven to 400°F for 10 minutes. Line a cookie sheet with aluminium foil and spray with vegetable-oil spray. Spread the fava beans evenly without crowding, and roast them for 15 minutes, or until they turn slightly brown. Remove from the oven and set aside.

4. In a large bowl, mix the peanuts, fava beans, and mung beans. Sprinkle the fried curry leaves (or the mint leaves), salt, cayenne pepper, and garlic powder (if using), over the mixture, and toss it well.

Transfer to a serving bowl and enjoy with your favorite drink. Save the leftover mix in an airtight jar.

Lentils

Soups and stews are a regular way lentils are enjoyed around the world, possibly because lentils hold their shape in this form. Few, if any, restaurants leave lentil soup out of their menu. Boiled lentils, dressed with vinaigrette, are also enjoyed as salads. More and more high-end restaurants are serving lentils, especially the less familiar French and Beluga types, as sides to entrées, an indication that lentils are increasingly being recognized as the tasty and nutritious food they are.

Lentil and Lemon Soup

SERVES 4

2 tablespoons olive oil

1 medium onion, chopped

2 stalks celery, chopped

1 yellow or orange bell pepper, sliced thin

1 cup red or brown lentils, rinsed and drained

4 cups of vegetable stock

1 lemon, juiced and zest (the peel) grated

1 teaspoon ground cumin

Salt and pepper to taste

1 tablespoon chopped parsley

1. In a medium-size soup pot, sauté the onion and celery in olive oil over medium heat until they have softened; add the bell pepper and cook for 2 minutes.

2. Add the lentils, stock, lemon zest, cumin, salt, and pepper. Cook for 30 minutes.

3. Lower the heat and let the soup simmer for another 30 minutes. Remove from heat and add the lemon juice. Sprinkle with parsley.

Serve the soup hot. With a salad on the side, this soup makes a nourishing meal.

French Green Lentils with Sun-Dried Tomatoes

SERVES 4

1 cup green lentils, rinsed and drained

1 cup sun-dried tomatoes, diced

1 cup white wine (use what you drink, not what is sold as cooking wine)

1 red onion, chopped

2 cloves of garlic, finely chopped

1 celery stalk, leaves removed and sliced thin

1 tablespoon chopped basil

2 tablespoons olive oil

1 teaspoon sugar

Salt and pepper to taste

1 tablespoon of crème fraiche (optional)

1. Heat the oil in a soup pot over medium heat. Sauté the onion and garlic in a pan until the onions are soft.

2. Add the lentils, celery, and sun-dried tomatoes to the pot. Add the sugar and water and let simmer for 30 minutes. Add the wine in the last 3 minutes of the simmer.

3. Remove from heat. Add the chopped basil, salt, and pepper, to taste.

Ladle the lentils into serving bowls and top with a spoonful of crème fraiche on each serving, if desired.

Serve with a crusty piece of bread on the side.

Red Lentils with Zucchini

SERVES 6

3 tablespoons vegetable oil

1 tablespoon melted butter

1 large onion, chopped

1 piece of ginger, peeled and minced

5 cloves garlic, finely chopped

1 green chili pepper, seeded and finely chopped

$1/2$ teaspoon ground turmeric

$1/4$ teaspoon ground cayenne pepper

1 teaspoon ground cumin

1 pound red lentils, cleaned, rinsed, and drained

4 cups water

1 pound zucchini, peeled and cut into $1/2$-inch cubes

1 cup chopped tomatoes

2 tablespoons chopped cilantro leaves

$1/2$ teaspoon salt or to taste

1. Heat the oil and butter in a pot over medium heat. Add the onion, ginger, garlic, green chili pepper, turmeric, cayenne pepper, and cumin. Cook until onions are soft, about 2–3 minutes, stirring frequently to prevent the mix from sticking to the bottom of the pot. Add the lentils and water and bring to a boil. Lower heat, cover, and simmer for 15–20 minutes or until lentils are tender, but not fully cooked.

2. Add the zucchini, tomatoes, and half the chopped cilantro leaves. Cook for 10 more minutes, or until vegetables are soft and a lentil squeezed between your thumb and index finger crumbles easily. Add salt and the remaining cilantro. Stir well and remove from the heat.

Serve warm with white or brown rice or whole-wheat bread.

Beluga Lentil Salad with Couscous and Baby Spinach

This is a variation of a salad I enjoyed at a restaurant in Canada. It is easy to make and is packed with a punch, nutritionally.

SERVES 6

$1/2$ cup beluga lentils, cleaned, rinsed, and drained

1 teaspoons olive oil

4 cups vegetable broth

1 cup couscous, uncooked

2 cups fresh baby spinach, triple rinsed, drained, and blotted dry

Ingredients for dressing

2 large lemons, juiced

$1/4$ cup champagne vinegar

2 tablespoons olive oil

2 teaspoons Dijon mustard

1 teaspoon sugar

$1/2$ teaspoon white pepper

1 avocado, peeled and sliced, for garnish

$1/4$ seedless watermelon, sliced into 2" pieces, for garnish

1. Place the lentils with 2 cups of vegetable broth in a pot and bring to a boil. Let boil for about 5 minutes, then reduce heat, cover, and simmer for 15–20 minutes or until tender. Avoid overcooking lentils, as they will get mushy.

2. Once lentils are done, remove from heat, drain fully, then season lightly with salt and pepper. Allow to cool for 5–10 minutes

3. While the lentils are cooking, add olive oil and remaining 2 cups of vegetable broth to a small pot, cover, and bring to a boil. Remove from heat and pour in the couscous. Stir the mixture well and keep it covered for 5 minutes, or until ready to use.

4. Combine all the dressing ingredients in a bowl, whisk the mixture, and set aside.

5. In a salad bowl, combine the cooked lentils, couscous, baby spinach, and pour in the dressing and mix well. Sprinkle salt and pepper. Let it cool and refrigerate until ready to serve, or serve at room temperature.

6. When ready to eat, arrange the salad on serving plates, and place the garnish on top.

Serve by itself or as a side with meat or fish.

Lentil and Barley Stew

SERVES 4

2 tablespoons vegetable or olive oil

1 bay leaf

1 medium onion, chopped

4 cloves garlic, minced

2 carrots, peeled and sliced

2 celery stems without leaves, sliced

1 cup mushrooms, sliced

1 cup brown lentils, rinsed and drained

1 cup pearl barley, uncooked

4 cups vegetable broth

1 cup water, plus more as needed

1 teaspoon freshly ground black pepper

Salt to taste

1 tablespoon chopped fresh basil

1. Heat the oil in a large soup pot over medium heat; add the bay leaf, onion, and garlic. Cook for 2 minutes and stir in carrots, celery, and mushrooms. Cook for 5 minutes or until vegetables are tender.

2. Add lentils, barley, vegetable broth, 1 cup water, and bring to a boil. Lower heat, cover, and simmer for 20–25 minutes, or until the lentils and barley are fully cooked, checking intermittently to see if more water is needed.

3. Season with salt, pepper, and basil leaves, and remove from heat.

Serve warm with a salad on the side to make a meal.

Lentils with Mung Bean Sprouts

SERVES 4

1 pound lentils (any type), rinsed and drained

4 tablespoons vegetable oil

3 dry whole red chili pepper pods

1 medium onion, peeled and sliced into rings

4 garlic cloves, finely chopped

1-inch piece of ginger, peeled and minced

2 large carrots, peeled and sliced

1 stem of celery without the leaves, sliced thin

1 green bell pepper, seeded and sliced into thin strips

1 red bell pepper, seeded and sliced into thin strips

1 large tomato, sliced into wedges

$1/2$ teaspoon salt or to taste

2 tablespoons freshly chopped basil

4 ounces of mung bean sprouts, freshly sprouted or purchased*

*Asian cooking incorporates bean sprouts in many of its dishes, main courses
as well as appetizers. Sprouting enhances the nutritional value of the legume.
If you are not ready to sprout your own beans, they are available in Asian
markets and, increasingly, in many larger grocery stores.*

1. Place lentils in a pot and cover with enough water so it is standing at least 1 inch above the lentils. Bring to a boil over medium-high heat. Lower heat and simmer for 20–25 minutes or until the lentils are soft. Remove from heat and set aside.

2. Heat oil in a skillet over medium heat; add the red chili pods, and fry for 30 seconds. Add onion, garlic, and ginger, cook for 2 minutes. Stir in chopped carrots and celery, cook another 2 minutes, then add bell peppers and tomato wedges. Continue cooking 1 more minute, leaving the bell peppers partially cooked and crisp. Stir in cooked lentils and mix well.

3. Season with salt and chopped basil leaves. Remove from heat and discard the chili pepper pods.

Serve warm over a bed of rice or quinoa.

Summary

People were initially introduced to novel foods by the development of agriculture, and later through technologies brought about by the industrial revolution, for which the human genome had little evolutionary experience. These novel foods, many of which are highly processed, include cereals, meats, dairy products, refined sugars, oils, and alcohol, which make up a significant proportion of the contemporary diet, but would have contributed little or nothing to pre-industrial or pre-agricultural diets. There is, for example, no precedent in human evolution for the ever-increasing amounts of refined sugar being consumed now. And the introduction of high-fructose corn syrup (HFCS) to replace sugar as a cheaper alternative in food processing and as a sweetener in beverages has been implicated in the steady and rapid increase in rates of overweight and obesity in the United States.

Regular consumption of increasingly larger portions of food and an associated sedentary lifestyle have resulted in rising rates of heart disease, adult-onset diabetes, cancer, and other chronic conditions referred to as *diseases of civilization*. While the prevalence of these diseases is higher in the United States and many Western European countries, they are also rising in other countries where diets are trending toward those of the West. These Western-style diets basically consist of more meat, dairy products, processed foods, and refined sugars, and less fruits, vegetables, legumes, and nuts. In

147

different countries and regions across the world, there is mounting evidence, brought to light by vast amounts of scientifically collected data over decades, that deviating from a predominantly plant-based diet is a major factor in the development of these diseases of civilization. When traditionally legume-eating populations switch to Western-type diets with more animal-based foods, and less plant-based foods, they lose the advantages they enjoyed of having better health, and instead, much like their Western counterparts, increasingly succumb to rising rates of obesity and the accompanying chronic diseases.

This association between diet and disease is incremental, as seen in the case of the Mediterranean diet in Greece, where even a modest increase in adherence to the traditional diet was associated with a significant reduction in overall mortality. This is a powerful lesson to learn from, and lends strong support to the recommendation by the USDA and other organizations to eat a diet consisting primarily of plant-based foods—fruits, legumes, nuts, seeds, vegetables, and whole grains—and less meat, processed foods, and sweets. Stated another way, it is good not to rely predominantly on animal foods for your nutrients, protein in particular, when it is more prudent to get them from a mix of well-diversified sources.

It has long been known that beans, peas, and lentils are much more than poor man's meat. They have remained a staple for thousands of years in many regions of the world. Legumes have even been credited with saving civilizations from perishing. Dry beans, peas, and lentils are a lean protein, complex-carbohydrate, high-fiber food loaded with many essential vitamins, minerals, and phytochemicals. They are low in fat, and contain no saturated fats. As plant-based food, legumes not only have no cholesterol in them, but also contain a generous amount of soluble fiber that acts as a scavenger to rid the body of circulating LDL (the bad cholesterol). The insoluble fiber in legumes is also beneficial as it aids in moving the bowels regularly. The low-glycemic index of legumes prevents the peaks and valleys (rapid rise and fall) in blood-sugar levels, which is detrimental to health, and also serves as a powerful tool to curb hunger between meals by being slow to empty out of the stomach, thereby keeping you feeling satisfied longer. In addition, legume plants' nitrogen-fixing property causes soil enrichment, making the crop eco-friendly as it contributes to sustainable farming. These are proven science-based facts about legumes that attest to their being a super food, a label reserved for the most potent, nutrient-rich foods having little to no ill effects and many important health benefits.

Legumes are not a boring food only good for making one or two dishes. As detailed in Chapter 5 and demonstrated in recipes in Chapter 7, they are very versatile foods that lend themselves to many tasty, flavorful, and aesthetically appealing dishes, from hors d'oeuvres, salads, and soups, to desserts around the world. The same legume may be used as a thick soup in Greece, a salty snack in China, a spicy curried dish in India, crunchy fritters in Nigeria, and an ice-cream ingredient in the Philippines. Yes, you do need to plan ahead if you don't want to eat them out of a can. But using the quick-soak method can reduce their soaking time, and pressure-cooking can cut the cooking time in half or more. Legumes can and should be a welcome addition to *any* healthy, well-balanced diet and not be looked upon as a special occasion food that takes a long time to prepare and is not worth the trouble.

All the known health and nutritional facts about legumes make having them on the plate regularly worth the small inconvenience associated with preparation and cooking. And any minor discomfort from flatulence, caused by indigestible complex sugars in legumes, can be countered or minimized by steps taken to reduce gas production during the preparation, cooking, and eating of legumes. These include such measures as bringing dry beans and peas to a quick boil before soaking, and changing the water a few times during soaking. Seasoning food during cooking with known anti-flatulence agents like fennel and ginger helps, as does ingesting enzyme-based compounds like Beano that prevent and/or neutralize gas before eating meals. In light of new or useful information, it is not uncommon for people to change the way something is thought about. A great deal of science-based information is now available on the diet/disease connection that should help reframe the thinking about foods in general, and super foods like legumes in particular.

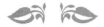

Recommended Reading

Bittman, M, Witschonke, A. *How to Cook Everything Vegetarian: Simple Meatless Recipes for Great Food.* Hoboken, NJ: Wiley Publishing, Inc., 2007.

Campbell, TC, Campbell, TM II. *The China Study.* Dallas, TX: BenBella Books, Inc., 2006.

Castelli, WP, Griffin, GC. *The New Good Fat Bad Fat: Lower Your Cholesterol & Reduce Your Odds of a Heart Attack.* Tucson, AZ: Fisher Books, 1997.

Colwell, L. "Brilliant Beans!" *New Vegetarian & Natural Health.* 25, Nov 2002, 39.

Crowey, A. "Spilling the Beans on Snacking Trends." *Food Magazine.* Apr 2009, 10–11.

Dragonwagon, C. *Bean by Bean: A Cookbook.* New York, NY: Workman Publishing, 2011.

Food Marketing Institute. *Trends in the United States: Consumer Attitudes and the Supermarket.* Washington, DC: FMI, 1992.

Fraley, A. "For Health, Legumes Hard to Beat." *Grit.* 120, Dec 2002, 22.

Giugliano, D, Sedge, M, Sepe, J. *The Mediterranean Diet: Its Origins and Myths.* Reddick, FL: Idelson-Gnocchi, 2000.

Haber, B. "The Mediterranean Diet: A View from History." *American Journal of Clinical Nutrition.* 66, 1997, 1053S–1057S.

Haber, D. *What Color Is Your Diet?* New York, NY: Regan Books, 2001.

Harvey, BS. "Meat or Beans: What Will You Have? Part 1I: Beans." *Harvard Men's Health Watch.* 15, Mar 2011, 4–6.

Hess, MA. "Taste: The Neglected Nutrition Factor." *American Journal of Dietetic Association.* 97 (2), 1997, S205–S207.

Hu, FB. "Plant-Based Foods and Prevention of Cardiovascular Disease: An Overview." *American Journal of Clinical Nutrition.* 78, 2003, 544S–551S.

Hurley, J, Lieberman, B. "Leapin' Legumes! Beans Come out of the Cupboard." *Nutrition Action Healthletter.* 31(7) Sept 2004, 12–13.

Jain, MG, Hislop, GT, Howe, GR, et al. "Plant Foods, Antioxidants, and Prostate Cancer Risk: Findings from Case-Control Studies in Canada." *Nutritional Cancer.* 34, 1999, 173–184.

James, PT, Leach, R, Kalamara, E, et al. "The Worldwide Obesity Epidemic." *Obesity Research.* 9, 2001, 228S–233S.

Jenkins, DJA, Wolever, T, Taylor, R, et al. "Exceptionally Low Blood Glucose Response to Dried Beans: Comparison with Other Carbohydrate Foods." *British Medical Journal.*281, 1980,:578–580.

Key, TJ, Schatzkin, A, Willett, WC, et al. "Diet, Nutrition, and Prevention of Cancer." *Public Health Nutrition* 7. (1A), 2004, 187–200.

Kiple, KF, Ornelas, KC, eds. *The Cambridge World History of Food, Vol 1.* Cambridge, MA: Cambridge University Press, 2000.

Krebs-Smith, SM, Kantor, LS. "Choose a Variety of Fruits and Vegetables Daily: Understanding the Complexities." *Journal of Nutrition.* 131, 2001. 487S–501S.

Lino, M. "The Thrifty Food Plan, 1999: Revisions of the Market Baskets." *Family Economics and Nutrition Review.* 13, 2001, 50–63.

Ludwig, DS. "Clinical Update: The Low-Glycemic-Index Diet." *The Lancet.* 369, 2007, 890–892.

Messina, MJ, Wu, AH. "Perspectives on the Soy-Breast Cancer Relation." *American Journal of Clinical Nutrition.* 89, 2009, 1673S–1679S.

Nestle, M, ed. *Food Politics: How the Food Industry Influences Nutrition and Health, 1st Ed.* Los Angeles, CA: University of California Press, Ltd., 2002.

Ross, T, Trafford, J. *Easy Beans: Fast and Delicious Beans, Pea, and Lentil Recipes, 2nd ed.* Vancouver, BC: Big Ben Publishing, 2003.

Schmid, RF. *Traditional Foods Are Your Best Medicine: Improving Health and Longevity with Native Nutrition.* Rochester, NY: Healing Arts Press, 1987.

Spiller, G, Spiller, M. *What's with Fiber: Enjoy Better Health with a High-Fiber, Plant-Based Diet.* Laguna Beach, CA: Basic Health Publications, Inc. 2005.

Stone, G, Campbell, CT. *Forks Over Knives: The Plant-Based Way to Health (eds).* New York, NY: Experiment Publishing, 2011.

Taubes, G. *Good Calories, Bad Calories.* New York, NY: Knopf, 2007.

Webb, D. "New, Natural Ways to Fight Cholesterol." *Prevention.* 53 (9), Sep 2001,: 68–69.

Welland, D. "Good Nutrition Is Full of Beans (and Peas and Lentils)." *Environmental Nutrition.* 21, 1998, 2–4.

Willett, WC, Stampfer, MJ. "Rebuilding the Food Pyramid." *Scientific American Special Edition.* 16 (4), 2006, 12–21.

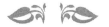

References

Chapter 1

1. Albala, K. *Beans Through History and Around the World*. London, UK: Berg Publishers, 2007.

2. Jenner, A. *The Amazing Legume: Cooking with Lentils, Beans, & Peas*. New York, NY: Woodstock, 1989, 9.

Chapter 2

1. Glanz, K, Basil, M, Maibach, E, et al. "Why Americans eat what they do: taste, nutrition, cost, convenience, and weight control concerns as influences on food consumption." *Journal of the American Dietetic Association*. 98, 1998, 1118–1126.

2. Palmer, S. "Loving Legumes for all the right reasons: health, flavor and value." *Environmental Nutrition*. 33 (4) April 2010, 1–3.

3. U.S. Department of Health and Human Services and U.S. Department of Agriculture. *Dietary Guidelines for Americans, 2010*. www.healthierus.gov/dietaryguidelines. Retrieved 2/21/2011.

4. Peters, MT, Schatzkin, A, Gierach, LG, et al. "Physical Activity and Postmenopausal Breast Cancer Risk in the NIH-AARP Diet and Health Study." *Cancer Epidemiology, Biomarkers & Prevention*. 18(1), January 2009, 289–302.

5. Simon, BH. "Meat or beans: What will you have? Part 1: Meat." *Harvard Men's Health Watch*. 15, Feb 2011, 1–3.

6. Simon, BH. "Meat or beans: What will you have? Part 1I: Beans." *Harvard-Men'sHealth Watch*. 15, Mar 2011) 4–6.

Chapter 4

1. Kiple, KF, Ornelas, KC, eds. *The Cambridge World History of Food*. Cambridge, MA: Cambridge University Press, 2000.

2. Gill, T, James, TP, Lakin, V. "Obesity: Preventing and Managing the Global Epidemic." *World Health Organization Technical Report Series*, 894, 2000.

3. Trichoppulou, A, Costacou, T, Bamia, C, et al. "Adherence to a Mediterranean Diet and Survival in a Greek Population." *New England Journal of Medicine*, 348, 2003, 2599–2608.

4. Keys, A, Menotti, M, Karvonen, J. et al. "The diet and 15-year death rate in the Seven Countries Study." *American Journal of Epidemiology.* 24, 1986, 903–915.

5. National Statistical Service of Greece. *Household Budget Surveys (HBS).* In Statistical Study on the Natural Movement of the Greek Population. Athens: National Statistical Service of Greece, 2008.

6. International Obesity Task Force. "Obesity Prevention: the case for action." *International Journal of Obesity.* 26(3), Mar 2002, 425–436.

7. Renaud, S, Lorgeril, DM, Delaye, J, et al. "Cretan Mediterranean diet for prevention of coronary heart disease." *American Journal of Clinical Nutrition.* 61(6), Jun 1995, 1360–1367.

8. Trichoppoulou, A, Costacou, T, Bamia, C, et al. "Adherence to a Mediterranean diet and survival in a Greek population." *The New England Journal of Medicine.* 348, 2003, 2599–2608.

9. Moreno, LA, Sarria, A, Popkin, BM. "The Nutrition Transition in Spain: a European Mediterranean country." *European Journal of Clinical Nutrition.* 56, 2002, 992–1002.

10. Zizza, C, Gerrior, S. "Trends in Availability of Foods and Nutrients: A comparison between the United States and Italy 1961–92." *Family Economics and Nutrition Review.* 12(1), Jan 1999, 26–42.

11. Correa-Leite, ML, Nicolosi, A, Cristina, S, et al. "Dietary and nutritional patterns in an elderly rural population in Northern and Southern Italy: II. Nutritional profiles associated with food behaviors." *European Journal of Clinical Nutrition.* 57, 2003, 1522–1529.

12. Sichieri, R. "Is fat intake important in the public health control of obesity?" *American Journal of Clinical Nutrition.* 72, 2000, 203–204.

13. Sichieri, R. "Dietary Patterns and their Associations with Obesity in the Brazilian City of Rio de Janeiro." *Obesity Research.* 10(1), Jan 2002, 42–48.

14. Campbell, TC, Chen, J. "Diet and chronic degenerative diseases: Perspectives from China." *American Journal of Clinical Nutrition.* 59, 1994. 1153–1161.

15. Shetty, PS. "Nutrition transition in India." *Public Health Nutrition.* 5(1), Jan 2002, 175–182.

16. Gopalan, C. "Obesity in the urban middle class." *Nutritional Foundation of India Bulletin.* 19, 1998, 1–4.

17. Food and Agriculture Organization (FAO) and World Health Organization (WHO). "Fats and Oils in Human Nutrition: Report of a joint expert consultation." *FAO Food and Nutrition Papers.* 57, 1994.

18. Gopinath, N, Chadha, SL, Jain, P, et al. "An epidemiological study of obesity in adults in the urban population of Delhi." *Journal of the Association of Physicians of India.* 42, 1994, 212–215.

19. Dharundhar, NV, Kulkarni, PR. "Prevalence of obesity in Bombay." *International Journal of Obesity and Related Metabolic Disorders.* 16, 1992, 367–375.

20. Zagar, AM, Masoodi, SR, Laway, BA, et al. "Prevalence of obesity in adults -an epidemiological study from Kashmir Valley of Indian subcontinent." *Journal of the Association of Physicians of India.* 48, 2000, 1170–1174.

21. Bourne, LT, Langerhoven, ML, Steyn, K, et al. "Nutrient intake in the urban African population of the Cape Peninsula, South Africa. The Brisk Study." *Central African Journal of Medicine.* 39(12), Dec 1993, 238–247.

22. Bourne, LT, Estelle, V, Lambert, S, et al. "Where does the black population of South Africa stand on the nutrition transition? *Public Health Nutrition.* 5(1A), Jan 2002, 157–162.

23. Institute of Medicine of the National Academies. "Dietary fats: total fat and fatty acids." In: Dietary reference intakes for energy, carbohydrate, fiber, fatty acids, cholesterol, protein, and amino acids (macronutrients). Washington DC: *The National Academy Press,* 2002.

24. Whitaker, JW. "Feedlot empire: beef cattle feeding in Illinois and Iowa, 1840–1900." Ames, IA: *The Iowa State University Press.* 1975.

25. Popkin, BM, Siega-Riz, AM, Pamela, SH, et al. "Where's the Fat? Trends in U.S. Diets 1965–1996." *Preventive Medicine.* 32(30), Mar 2001, 245–254.

26. Simon, BH. "Meat or beans: What will you have? Part 1: Meat." *Harvard Men's Health Watch.* 15 (7), Jul 2011, 1–3.

27. Samara, JN, Popkin, BM. "Patterns and Trends in Food Portion Sizes, 1977–1998." *Journal of the American Medical Association (JAMA).* 289(4), Apr 2003, 450–453.

28. Glanz, K, Basil, M, Maibach, E, et al. "Why Americans eat what they do: Taste, nutrition, cost, convenience, and weight control concerns as influences on food consumption." *Journal of the American Dietetic Association.* 98, 1980, 1118–1126.

Chapter 6

1. Green, A. *The Bean Bible: A Legumaniac's Guide to Lentils, Peas, and Every Edible Bean on the Planet!* Philadelphia, PA: Running Press, 2000.

Chapter 7

1. Green, A. *Beans: More than 200 Delicious, Wholesome Recipes from Around the World.* Philadelphia: Running Press, 2004.

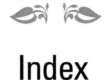

Index

Achiote, 102, 103, 106

Adzuki Bean Mango Stir-Fry with Cilantro, Lime, and Coconut Sauce, 128–129

Adzuki Beans with Baby Bok Choy, 129–130

Aflatoxin, 47

Agriculture, 31, 147

ALA, 26, 66

Albala, Ken, 6

Algae, 26

Alphagalactosidase, 90

Alpha-linolenic acid (ALA). *See* ALA.

Amazing Legume, The (Jenner), 8

American Association of Retired Persons (AARP), 16, 55

American Heart Association, 29

Amino acids, 2, 15, 21–22

Anti-inflammatories, 65

Antioxidants, 19, 23, 65, 67, 78

Arginine, 82

Arteries, 23

Arthritis, 27

Asafetida, 90, 124

Atherosclerosis, 21, 29

Authentic Louisiana Red Beans and Rice, 98

Bacteria, *rhizobium,* 3

Baghalee Popo, 114

Bagiana, 113

Baingan barta, 118

Baked beans, 112

Baking soda, 88

Barley, 145

Basal metabolic rate (BMR), 25

Beano, 89, 90, 149

Beans, 7, 42, 148

   adzuki, 75–76, 128–130

   black, 10, 64–66, 103–107, 110

   black turtle, 66–67, 103

   canned/pre-cooked, 3, 12, 62, 70, 89–90

   cannellini/white kidney, 68, 107–111

   common, 5, 61–68

   diversity of, 7

   dry, 3, 7, 9–10, 61–68

   fava/broad, 5, 69–70, 113–117, 140

   garbanzo. *See* Chickpeas.

   lima, 5, 70–72, 93, 118–120

   Mesoamerican, 7

   mung, 74–75, 91, 122–127, 140, 146

   pinto/mottled, 63–64, 100–103

   red/kidney, 61–63, 96–100, 110

white/navy, 67–68, 108–109, 112–113

See also Black-eyed peas; Chickpeas; Lentils; Peanuts; Peas; Soybeans; Split peas.

Beans (Green), 93, 107

Beans Through History and Around the World (Albala), 6

Beantown. See Boston, Massachusetts.

Beer, 23, 37

Beluga Lentil Salad with Couscous and Baby Spinach, 144–145

Betel nuts, 89

Bile, 21, 80

Bitterness, 113

Black-eyed peas, 76–77, 93, 130–133

Black-Eyed Peas and Baby Kale Salad, 132–133

Black-Eyed Peas with Pork and Greens, 131–132

Blood sugar, 14, 22–23, 24, 66, 79, 80, 86, 148

BMI. *See* Body mass index (BMI).

Body fat, 20

Body mass index (BMI), 20, 42, 45–46, 53

Boil and soak method
quick, 87, 89, 93, 95, 103, 149
slow, 87, 95

Bok choy, 129

Bolo-Rei, 114

Boston, Massachusetts, 4, 6, 112

Boston Baked Beans, 112–113

Bowel movements, 14, 23, 80, 148

Brazilian Food Pyramid, 64

Burritos, 100, 103

Butyric acid, 66

Calcium, 25

Caldo de frijol, 104

Calories, 25–26, 28, 35, 50

Campbell, Colin, 45

Cancers, 17, 27, 32, 36, 38, 46, 55, 58, 65, 80
breast, 46–47
colon, 55
liver, 47

Cannellini Bean and Vegetable Soup, 109

Caparrones, 96

Cape Town, South Africa, 51–52

Carbohydrates, 24, 40, 42, 47, 52, 70, 148

Cardiovascular disease. *See* Heart diseases.

Carom seeds, 90

Cells, 19, 23

Cellulose, 14

Cereals, 33

Channa masala. *See* Chickpea Curry (Channa Masala).

Chapatti, 96

Chard, 111

Cheese, 39
Parmesan, 111
Pecorino Romano, 113, 114

Cheeseburgers, 56

Chen, Junshi, 45

Chicken, 105

Chickpea Curry (Channa Masala), 135–136

Chickpeas, 5, 78–79, 116, 133–137

Chili con carne, 62, 96, 99–100

Chinese Academy of Preventive Medicine, Institute of Nutrition and Food Hygiene, 44

Cholesterol, 14, 20–21, 28, 38, 46, 47, 48, 49, 77, 148
high-density lipoprotein (HDL), 21, 29
low-density lipoprotein (LDL), 21, 22, 27–28, 29, 73, 82, 148

Chutneys, 125, 135

Cilantro, 128
Cilantro, Lime and Coconut Sauce, 129
Coconuts, 128
Colon, 79
Continuing Survey of Food Intake by Individuals, 56
Copper, 14
Corn, 3, 40
Cosenza, Italy, 41
Couscous, 144
Crepes. See Dosas.
Crop rotation, 3
Crops, 5
    New World, 7
    Old World, 70
Croutons, 108
Cuban Black Bean Soup with Smoked Turkey, 106–107
Cuisines
    American, 139
    Asian, 88, 91, 120, 122, 128, 139, 146
    Basque, 100
    Brazilian, 103
    Creole, 96, 98, 103
    Cuban, 103, 106
    Egyptian, 114, 115
    Indian, 88, 94, 96–97, 118, 122, 133, 134, 135, 138, 139
    Indonesian, 122
    Italian, 113, 114
    Japanese, 128
    Korean, 114
    Latin American, 103
    Mediterranean, 114
    Mexican, 110
    Middle Eastern, 114, 133
    Moroccan, 138
    New England, 112
    Philippines, 122
    Puerto Rican, 102

Tex-Mex, 96, 99–100, 103, 105
    Sichuan, 114
    South American, 103
    Southern, 130
    See also Diet.
Culture, Southern, 77
Curried Red Kidney Beans (Rajma Dal), 96–97
Curries, 94, 96, 135–136
Curry, 94, 96
    leaves, 123
    powder, 94

Dairy products, 37, 38, 39, 40, 50, 58
Dal, 96, 138
Daniel (Biblical character), 8
Desserts, 28
DHA, 26
Diabetes, adult-onset, 32, 48, 58
Diet, 2, 16–17, 23, 25, 26, 28, 31–33, 41–42, 47, 48, 52, 57, 147–148
    American/Western, vii–viii, 3, 9–10, 26–27, 43, 53–58
    Asia, 3, 10, 74, 75, 88
    Brazil, 42–44
    China, 44–47
    Greece, 34–36
    India, 3, 6, 10, 47–51
    Italy, 38–42
    Mediterranean, 3, 7, 9, 16, 69, 148, 33–42
    plant-based, vii–viii, 2, 8–9, 16, 21, 37, 38, 44, 45, 46, 47, 59, 148
    rice and beans (Brazil), 42–44
    South Africa, 51–53
    South America, 3
    Spain, 36–38
    vegetarian, 46
    Westernization of, 32, 34, 42, 51, 53, 59

See also Cuisines.

Diet and Health Study, 55

Dietary Guidelines for Americans,
    2, 4, 16, 65

Digestion, 66, 80, 89

Diseases, chronic, 32–33, 46, 48, 51,
    51, 58, 59, 147–148
    See also Cancers; Diabetes;
    Heart diseases.

Dosas, 88, 124, 133

Dose response, 36

Doubanjiang, 114

Dove Creek, Colorado, 63

Earthenware, 90

Edamame, 120, 121

Edamame (Green Soybeans) with
    Garlic, 121

Education, 53

Eggplants, 118

Eggs, 39

EPA, 26

Es Kacang Hijau, 122

Esau (biblical character), 82

European Association for the Study
    of Obesity, 35

European Prospective Investigation
    of Cancer and Nutrition
    (EPIC), 36

Falafel, 116, 133

Falafel with Fava Beans and
    Chickpeas, 116–117

Farinata, 133

Fats, vii, 9, 14, 24, 35, 37, 39–40,
    42, 44, 45, 46, 48, 49, 50, 52,
    73, 82, 148
    monounsaturated, 28, 37
    polyunsaturated, 28–29, 37
    saturated, 27–28, 33, 53, 54
    trans, 29

Fava Bean Breakfast Spread, 115–116

Feijoda, 103

Fennel, 89, 90, 149

Fertilizers, 3

Fiber, 9, 14, 21, 22–23, 42, 46, 47,
    50, 55,–56, 68, 72, 75, 80, 148
    insoluble, 14, 22, 23, 66, 79, 148
    soluble, 14, 21, 22–23, 65, 75, 77,
    148

Figs, 40

Fish, 26, 29, 39

Flatulence, 12, 66, 87, 89–90, 93,
    103, 149

Flavonoids, 14, 23, 65

Flaxseeds, 26

Folate. *See* Folic acid.

Folic acid, 14, 65–66, 68, 70, 76, 85

Food and Agriculture Organization
    (FAO), 47, 49

*Food Guide for the Brazilian
    Population,* 64–65

Foods, 15, 24–25, 27, 31, 40, 52,
    56, 147
    animal-based, 22–22
    availability of, 49
    complementary to legumes, 2,
    15, 22
    costs of, 15
    fast, 57
    location of eating, 34, 54, 57–58
    plant-based, 22, 27, 50, 85–86
    portions, 32, 56
    processing of, 31–32
    taste of, 57

Free radicals, 19

French Green Lentils with Sun-
    Dried Tomatoes, 142

Fruits, 33, 35, 37, 38, 40, 50–51,
    52, 53, 56

Fufu, 71

Ful hamman, 114

Ful medame, 114

Ful rumi, 115

Gallo pinto, 103, 104
Gamma-linoleic acid (GLA), 26
Garlic, 121
Gas. *See* Flatulence.
Gastric emptying, 66
Genetics, 31, 32
GI. *See* Glycemic index (GI).
Ginger, 89, 90, 149
Ginisang Monggo, 122
GL. *See* Glycemic load (GL).
Glycemic index (GI), 23–24, 44,
    148
Glycemic load (GL), 23–24
Gochujang, 114
Golden Risotto with Baby Lima
    Beans and Red Pepper,
    119–120
Grains, 2, 3, 6, 22, 33, 39, 40, 41,
    50, 53, 56
Green, Aliza, 89
Greens, 90

Heart diseases, 2–3, 14, 16–17, 26,
    27, 29, 32, 33, 35, 38, 46, 48,
    58, 65–66
Hepatitis B, 47
Heterocyclic amines, 55
High fructose corn syrup (HFCS),
    31–32, 147
Homemade Curry, 94
Homocysteine, 14
Hopiang Munggo, 122
Hopkins, Anthony, 113
Hoppin' John, 130, 131
Hummus, 133, 137
Hunger, 23, 42, 66, 80, 148
Hydrogen, 29
Hydrogenation, 29
Hydrogen-cyanide gas, 118

Indian Mung Dal. *See* Saucy Mung
    Beans (Indian Mung Dal).

Industrialization, 48, 51, 52, 59
Inflammation, 17, 21, 23, 26, 26, 29,
    65
International Classification of
    Diseases (ICD-9), 58
International Obesity Task Force,
    35
Iron, 14, 25, 72
Isoflavones, 27, 80

Jacob (Biblical character), 82
Jenner, Alice, 8
Johannesburg, South Africa, 52

Kale, 131, 132
Keys, Ancel, 33

Legumes, viii, 1–4, 33, 34, 50, 56,
    61–86, 148–149
  accessibility of, 12
  blanching, 88
  cleaning, 87
  consumption by region, 9–10
  factors influencing consumption,
      11–12
  fermentation, 88, 120
  food value, 11, 13–17
  health benefits, 16–17
  history of consumption, 5–12,
      69–70
  nutrients of, 14–16, 63, 64,
      65–66, 68, 70, 72, 73, 75, 76,
      77, 78–79, 80, 82, 85–86
  preparation and cooking, 3, 12,
      87–89, 93, 95
  quality, 12
  recipes, 93–146
  refrigerating, 88, 92
  rural/urban consumption, of, 11
  seasoning, 88–89
  skins, 70, 80, 88, 89
  soaking, 3, 87, 88, 89, 149

socioeconomic status and, 10, 11,
     52, 53, 59
  sprouting, 74, 91–92
  stereotypes about, 4
  storing, 92
Lemons, 141
Lentil and Barley Stew, 145
Lentil and Lemon Soup, 141–142
Lentils, 3, 5, 15, 82–86, 88, 93,
     141–146, 148
  Beluga, 84–85, 144
  brown/green, 83
  French green, 83, 142
  red, 84, 143
Lentils with Mung Bean Sprouts,
     146
Life expectancy, 35, 36, 55, 59
Lima Beans with Roasted Eggplant,
     118
Limes, 128
Linoleic acid (LA), 26
Liver, 47
Louisiana, 96, 103
"Loving Legumes for All the Right
     Reasons" (article), 14–15
Lycopene, 27

Macronutrients, 24
Magnesium, 14, 66
Maize. See Corn.
Manganese, 14, 72
Mangoes, 128
Meat, 34, 35, 37, 38, 44, 53, 55, 58
  red, 8, 15, 16–17, 28, 39, 53–54,
     55
  processed, 17, 55
  white, 55
"Meat or Beans" (article), 17
Medical care, 38
Metabolic syndrome, 58
Metabolism, 25–26
Methionine, 15, 22

Mexican Bean Salad, 110
Micronutrients, 24–25, 75
Microwaves, 87
Milk. See Dairy products.
Minerals, 25, 79, 148
Mint Chutney, 135
Miso, 120
Molybdenum, 79
Moroccan Split Pea and Pumpkin
     Soup, 138–139
Morosy Cristianos, 103
Mortality. See Life expectancy.
Mung Bean and Rice Pilaf
     (Khichidi), 126–127
Mung Bean Crepes (Pesarattu or
     Dosa), 124
Mung dal, 122–123
Mushiness, 83, 84, 85, 89

N-nitroso compounds (NOC), 55
National Academy of Sciences,
     Committee on Diet, Nutrition,
     and Cancer, 33
National Institutes of Health (NIH),
     16, 55
National Research Council of Italy,
     41
National Statistical Service of
     Greece, 34
Nationwide Food Consumption
     Survey, 56
Natto, 120
New Year's Day, 77, 130, 131
Nitrates, 3
Nitrogen, 3
Nitrogen-fixation, 3, 149
Nitrosamines, 55
Noodles, cellophane, 122
Nutrition Foundation of India, 49

Obesity, 35, 37, 42–44, 45, 48,
     49–50, 53, 54, 58, 59, 147, 148

Oils, 39, 40
   annatto seed, 106
   olive, 35
   soybean, 121
   vegetable, 29
Oligosaccharides, 89
Omega-3 fatty acids, 26, 28, 65
Omega-6 fatty acids, 26–27, 28
Oxidation, 19
Oxidative stress, 17, 65

Pabellón criollo, 103
Pakoras, 133
Palmer, Sharon, 14–15
Pasta, 111
Pavia, Italy, 41
Peanut butter, 81, 139
Peanuts, 81–82, 139–141
Peas, 5, 148
   dried, 79–80
   See also Black-eyed peas;
   Chickpeas; Split peas.
Peppers, red, 119
Persimmons, 40
Phaseolus angularis. See Beans,
   adzuki.
Phaseolus vulgaris. See Beans,
   common.
Physical fitness/activity, 37, 46,
   48–49, 51
Phytochemicals, 27, 82, 148
Phytonutrients, 65
Pilafs, 126
Pineapples, 40
Pinto Beans and Yellow Rice,
   102–103
Pita Chips, 137
Populations, rural/urban, 11, 41–42,
   45, 48–50, 51–53
Pork, 131
Potassium, 14, 77
Potatoes, 39

Poultry, 28, 39
Pressure cooking, 87, 88, 89, 149
Proteins, 2, 3, 6, 14, 15, 21, 24, 39,
   45, 50, 52, 65, 66, 78, 80, 82,
   148
   complementary, 22
   complete, 2, 21–22, 73
Pulses. *See* Legumes.
Pumpkins, 138
Puy, France, 83

Quinoa, 104
Quinoa and Black Beans, 104

Rajma Dal. *See* Curried Red
   Kidney Beans (Rajma Dal).
Recommended daily values (DV),
   14, 15
Red bean paste, 128
Red beans and rice, 98, 100
Red Lentils with Zucchini, 143
Resveratrol, 82
Rice
   Arborio, 119
   yellow, 103
   white, 98, 126
Rosh Hashanah, 138

Saint Joseph Day, 69
Salad Dressing, 144
Salads, 110, 132, 133, 141, 144
Salt, 3, 12, 62, 70, 89
Satiation, 14, 23, 79, 86
Saucy Mung Beans (Indian Mung
   Dal), 122–123
Selenium, 14
Sicily, 69
Silence of the Lambs (movie), 113
Simon, Harvey, 17
Skordalia, 114
Slow-Cooker Pinto Beans, 101
Snacks, 54–55, 56–57, 139, 140

Sofrito, 102
Soft drinks, 56, 58
Soil, 3, 149
Sopa negra, 104
Soups, 103–104, 105, 106, 109, 111, 112, 113, 138–139, 141–142
South African Diet Consensus Panel, 52
Southwest Black Bean Chicken Soup, 105
Soy sauce, 120
Soybeans, 3, 15, 22, 72–73, 91, 120–121
Spanish Paradox, 38
Spices, 93, 94
Spicy Turkey Chili, 99–100
Spinach, 144
Split peas, 79–80, 88, 93, 138–139
Spreads, 28, 115
Sprouts, 74, 75, 85, 91–92, 146
Stews, 107, 141, 145
Sugar, 31, 35, 40, 41, 147
Super foods, 1–2, 16
Sweeteners, 40, 41

Tahini paste, 114, 117, 137
Tahini sauce, 117, 133
Tamari, 120
Tangshui, 122
Tea, 23, 27
Tempeh, 120
Tempura-Style Vegetables (Pakoras) with Mint Chutney, 134–135
Three-Legume Snack, 140–141
Tofu, 120–121
Tomato Chutney, 125–126
Tomatoes, 39, 40, 125, 142

Trans-fatty acid (TFA). See Fats, trans.
Triglycerides, 29
Turkey, 99, 106
Turmeric, 90
Tuscan Chard and Cannellini Bean Soup, 111
Tuscan White Bean Stew, 107–108
Twelfth Night, 70

U.S. Department of Agriculture (USDA), viii, 16, 148
U.S. Department of Health and Human Services (USDHHS), 2, 16
U.S. Food and Drug Administration (FDA), 29, 73, 92
United States Center for Nutrition Policy and Promotion, 38
University of North Carolina, 38, 54
Urbanization, 37, 48, 49, 51, 53

Vegetables, 35, 37, 40, 50–51, 52, 53, 56, 109
Vitamin A, 25
Vitamin B-complex, 25, 75
Vitamins, 24–25, 63, 65–66, 76, 85, 148

Water, 88, 89
Weight, viii, 1, 9, 20, 23, 25, 37, 42, 43, 51, 54, 57, 58, 59, 80, 86, 32
"Why American Eat What They Do" (article), 13
Wine, 2, 37

Zinc, 14
Zucchini, 143

About the Author

Swarna Moldanado has a Ph.D. in Nursing Science from the University of Illinois, Chicago, and has taught nursing and public health at colleges and universities in Illinois and California. Besides having a number of articles on the topics of public health and research methods in peer-reviewed journals, she has been awarded grants for projects in her areas of expertise, most particularly in the public health sector. Dr. Moldanado is a member of both the American Public Health Association and the California Public Health Association, North, and lives with her husband in Belmont, California.